Other books by this author:

To Be Invisible: Unveiling the Truth about Eating Disorders

Understanding Autism and Positive Behavioural Support

Level 3 Diploma for Children and Young People's Workforce: A comprehensive learner support guide

Dementia Care Certificate Levels 2 & 3

Leadership and Management in Health and Social Care and Children and Young Peoples' Services – The down-to-earth learner support guide

Dedicated to Amina and Timmy

DEMENTIA CARE CERTIFICATE

LEVELS 2 & 3

A Down-to-Earth Learning Companion for Health and Social Care

S.K. Porter-Brooks

CONTENTS

Introduction 11

Chapter 1: Dementia Awareness 13

    Defining Dementia 13

    Different Types of Dementia 16

        Different Areas of the Brain Affected by Dementia 16

        Alzheimer's Disease 18

        Vascular Dementia 18

        Pick's Disease/ Frontotemporal dementia 19

        Dementia with Lewy Bodies 21

        Creutzfeldt Jakob Disease (CJD) 22

        Huntingdon's Disease 23

        Dementia Syndrome or 'Mixed Dementia' 24

        HIV-Associated Dementia 24

    Statistics 26

        Prevalence of Different Types of Dementia 28

    Potential factors that contribute to the development of dementia – risk factors 29

    How dementia is Recognised and Other Conditions Might Be Mistaken for It 31

        Diagnostic Process 31

        The Importance of Ruling Out Other Conditions 33

        Why Early Diagnosis is Important 33

    Effects of Dementia on Cognitive Abilities 35

        Different Types of Memory 35

    Daily Life with Dementia 40

        Fluctuating Symptoms and the Importance of Effective Recording 48

        Relevance of the Social and Medical Model of Disability 49

        How Attitudes or Behaviour of Others Can Affect People with Dementia 51

  Is Dementia a Disability?..52

Chapter 2: The Person-Centred Approach to the Care and Support of Individuals with Dementia 53

  What are Person-Centred Values?...53

  Linking Ideas to Practice..57

  Being Proactive To Link People With Solutions 60

Chapter 3: Understand the Factors that can Influence Communication and Interaction with Individuals who have Dementia..63

  Introduction: Relationships and Communication 63

  Improving Communication for a Person with Dementia: Things to Consider Before you Speak 64

  Improving Communication for a Person with Dementia: Things to Consider While you Speak 69

  Communication with the Senses 72

  Validation Approach Versus Reality Orientation 77

Chapter 4: Understand Equality, Diversity and Inclusion in Dementia Care 79

  Definitions of Equality, Diversity, Anti-Discriminatory and Anti-Oppressive Practice...............83

   Why People with Dementia Can Experience Discrimination or Oppression 85

   How to Challenge Discriminatory and Oppressive Practice....................................88

  How Dementia Affects Different Types of People 89

   Younger People with Dementia 89

   People from Ethnic Minority Communities 90

   People with Learning or Physical Disabilities..91

  Extended Reading: Other Marginalised Groups Affected by Dementia 92

  Rights, Regulations and other Legal Protections 100

Chapter 5: Introduction Awareness of Models of Disability..................................104

  Models of Disability..104

  Psychosocial Model of Disability 106

  Development of Disability Models Through Time 107

Chapter 6: Understand the administration of medicines to individuals with dementia using a person-centred approach 109
- Medication for Reducing Dementia Symptoms 109
- Anti-Psychotics 112
- What are Psychotic Symptoms? 112
  - Hallucinations 113
  - Delusions 114
  - Thought disorders 117
  - Development of Anti-Psychotics: Risks and Benefits 117
- Antidepressants 119
- Anticonvulsants 119
- Anxiety 120
  - Treatments: 120
- Sleep Disturbances 121
  - Drug treatments: 121
- Pain 122
  - Treatment & Management of Pain 123
  - Medication Approaches 124
  - 'PRN' Medication 125
- Importance of Recording and Reporting Side-Effects 126
- Summary 127

Chapter 7: Understand mental well-being and mental health promotion 131
- Suggestions for a Collage Project 132
- Importance of Involvement and Engagement 134
- Strategies for Mental Health 136
  - No Health Without Mental Health (2011) 136
- Conclusion 138

References 139

INTRODUCTION

In many ways, the severity of the dementia problem, both in the UK and worldwide, is the price of modernity. It is a hefty price, however, and one that no one wants to have to pay, and is a burden for us all, but it seems we will have to live with it. We are living longer, and medical treatments are able to sustain our longevity in ways we could never have dreamed of in years gone by.

There are many dimensions to this problem, and literature on the topic often fails to encapsulate all of them. On one level, dementia is a very personal battle and in many ways a tragedy for the person who is affected and for all their friends and loved ones.

It is also a societal, and huge economic challenge. While it may seem pedantic to focus on statistics or forecasts about costs and workforce vacancies, these issues also have an impact on every single individual affected by dementia. Economic costs, challenges to the NHS and health and social care workforce, as well as pressures experienced by carers have a collective, and a very personal impact.

This book will strive to look at all of these different dimensions, while also providing a learning resource towards healthcare practitioners working towards Levels 2 & 3 Dementia Care Certificate. It is important that staff within the health and social care sector, understand the pressures and heartache that carers and loved ones of people with dementia, are going through.

As an independently published author, I have chosen to write a textbook that embraces the knowledge required both for the Level 2 and 3 Dementia Care Certificates. I decided to do this for many reasons. One reason, is a fact that we are all quite familiar with: wage rates for working in social care are poor, and if cost is a restriction to buying a book and following one's interests, then I'm all for finding ways to reduce costs. Secondly, many people working in social care these days have done so for a considerable amount of time, and have lots of experience of working in the sector, but may not have confidence when it comes to written work or formal coursework. Thirdly, many both new and experienced employees in the social care sector, have a deep interest and passion in understanding and delivering excellent quality of care for people with dementia. Therefore, in this book I decided to include some slightly more extended reading that is as applicable to the Level 2 as it is to the Level 3 certificate, and will be particularly pertinent to those wanting to progress from one level to the next.

You will notice the following symbol in places throughout the book: ✱ This symbol refers to information that is more directly relevant to the Level 3 Certificate, however can be treated as extended reading for those primarily working towards Level 2. This does not mean, however, that other information is not relevant to the Level 3.

I have decided not to refer to lots of course codes and 'assessment criteria', which can make a textbook look a bit like the Highway Code. However, you will I hope find in this book, all the information you need to learn and study towards both certificates.

CHAPTER 1: DEMENTIA AWARENESS

DEFINING DEMENTIA

In this section we will explore the definition of 'dementia'. As will become clear, there are many different types of dementia. Confusingly, some types of dementia display subtle differences in the nature of the initial symptoms, often leading to misdiagnosis or delays in diagnosis. A key element to any definition of 'dementia', is the fact that it is progressive, however. Ultimately, the differences in symptom expression between the varying types of dementia, become blurred over time.

In addition to this, there are four key areas of functionality that all tend to display some level of impairment, across all kinds of dementia, before a diagnosis can be made.

The person will manifest the following:

- A decline in memory
- A decline in reasoning and communication
- Changes in behaviour: decreased inhibition – e.g. saying inappropriate things; behaving inappropriately; becoming rigid in daily routines.
- A deterioration in everyday day-to-day activities: e.g. making a cup of tea.

In essence, the effects of dementia symptoms are evident in almost all aspects of functionality. This is conveyed by the acronym, 'MOST'.

This seems a suitable acronym in the way it brings into relief how the effects of dementia are so all-encompassing.

The acronym 'MOST', stands for:

TABLE 1 SYMPTOMS OF DEMENTIA USING THE ACRONYM 'MOST'

| M | Memory: | The individual will display deterioration in memory. It is important to note that there are different types of memory, which will be explored later in this book.

Different types of dementia will evince different effects on memory in the early stages. Although, as dementia is by nature progressive, the distinctions between the variable effects of different forms of dementia, become blurred in the later stages of the disease. |
|---|---|---|
| O | Orientation in Time and Space: | The individual may struggle to understand or remember where they are, what they are doing, what they are doing next.

They may also show deterioration in spatial awareness, and visual perception. |
| S | Social skills: | The individual may display personality changes. They may become more withdrawn and lacking in confidence. On the other hand, they may become disinhibited, and behave or speak with uncharacteristic aggressiveness. |
| T | Thinking: | The individual may present with or experience thought delusions, hallucinations, impairment in executive functioning, reasoning or communication abilities. |

Apply and Demonstrate

For your Certificate Award, you will need to demonstrate that you can write a definition for dementia.

Try to use the headings outlined in the table on the previous table and elaborate your answer with real-life examples.

Remember, never to use identifiable information relating to individual patients, and to respect their confidentiality.

DIFFERENT TYPES OF DEMENTIA

In the following section, we will explore some of the most common different types of dementia, and the risk factors that underlie them.

These include:

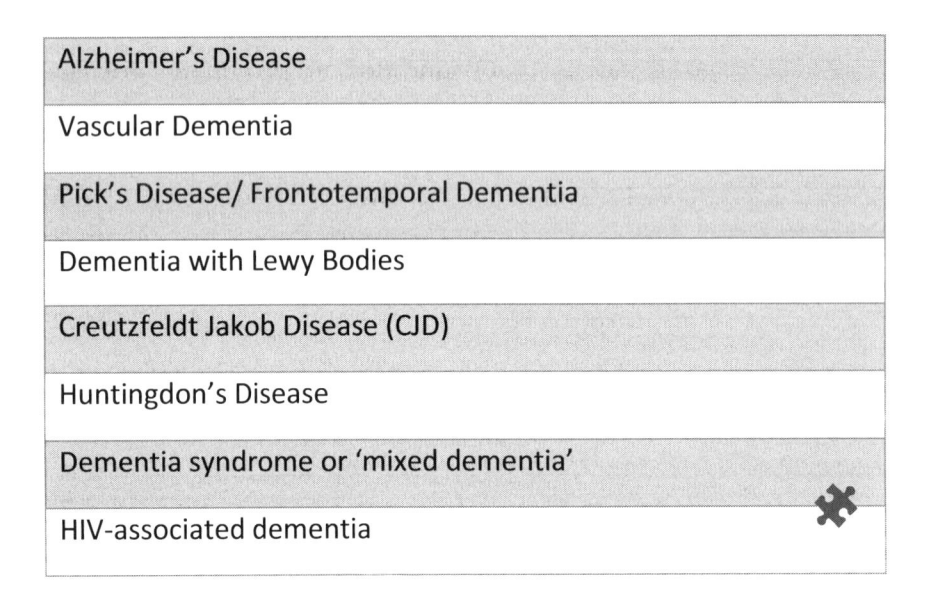

Alzheimer's Disease
Vascular Dementia
Pick's Disease/ Frontotemporal Dementia
Dementia with Lewy Bodies
Creutzfeldt Jakob Disease (CJD)
Huntingdon's Disease
Dementia syndrome or 'mixed dementia'
HIV-associated dementia

Different Areas of the Brain Affected by Dementia

With the progression of neuroscience, and pioneering brain imaging techniques, our understanding about how the brain works is much more advanced now than it ever was before, with further improvements occurring all the time.

We now understand that different symptoms will become manifest with dementia, depending on which areas of the brain have been affected.

This is particularly so, with vascular dementia, or multi-infarct dementia, where a number of minor isolated strokes have occurred. The effect of such mini-strokes, will depend on which area of the brain has been damaged, and the severity of the stroke.

TABLE 2 DIAGRAM OF THE CEREBRAL CORTEX/OUTSIDE OF THE BRAIN, HIGHLIGHTING THE SPECIFIC REGIONS[i]

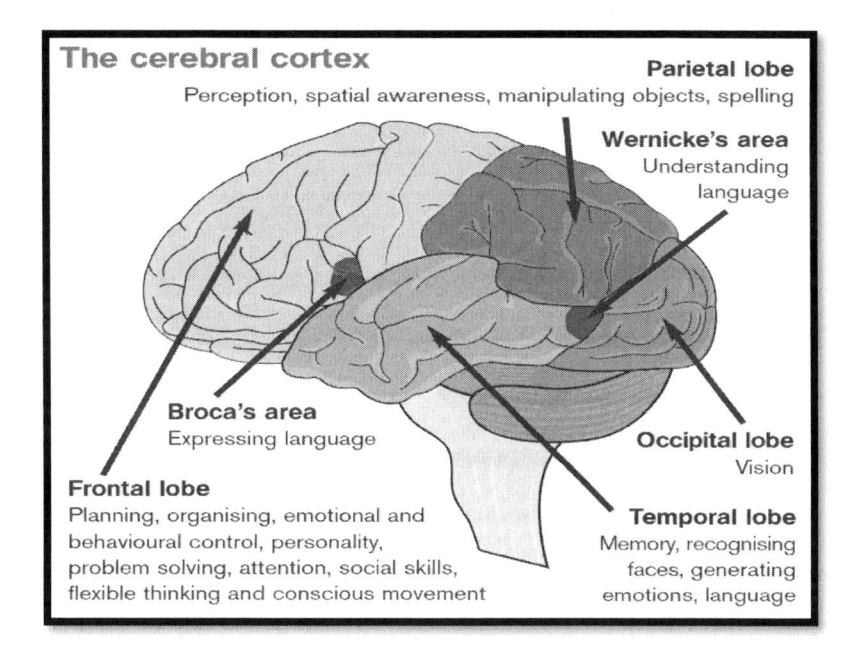

The cerebral cortex

- **Parietal lobe**: Perception, spatial awareness, manipulating objects, spelling
- **Wernicke's area**: Understanding language
- **Broca's area**: Expressing language
- **Occipital lobe**: Vision
- **Frontal lobe**: Planning, organising, emotional and behavioural control, personality, problem solving, attention, social skills, flexible thinking and conscious movement
- **Temporal lobe**: Memory, recognising faces, generating emotions, language

The table on the next page outlines the main different areas of the brain, and what their main area of functionality is:

Table 3 Functionality of Different Areas of the Brain

Frontal lobe	Planning, organising, emotional and behavioural control, personality, problem solving, attention, social skills, flexible thinking and conscious movement.
Temporal lobe	Memory, recognising faces, generating emotions, language.
Parietal lobe	Perception, spatial awareness, manipulating objects, spelling.
Wernicke's area	Understanding language
Broca's area	Expressing language
Occipital lobe	Vision

Alzheimer's Disease

Possibly the most well-known form of dementia, is Alzheimer's Disease. It was named after Alois Alzheimer, a German doctor.

The disease is characterised by the build-up of plaques around brain cells, which prevent them being able to communicate with each other.

There are thought to be a wide array of potential causes or risk factors behind the disease, for example: lifestyle; diet; general health; living environment. There is also a possible genetic link, and it has been found that those with the genetic variant are more susceptible to developing the disease.

Unfortunately, the term 'Alzheimer's disease' is so commonly known, that sometimes it is used misleadingly as a blanket term for all types of dementia. Many people associate all dementias with the symptoms commonly associated with Alzheimer's disease, even though the effects of different types of dementia are distinctively different, at least in the early stages.

Vascular Dementia

The vascular system is a network of veins and arteries that carry blood around the body. If it isn't working properly, then parts of the brain or body become deprived of blood and oxygen.

There are two main types of vascular dementia:

Infarct dementia	Caused by a stroke
Multi-infarct dementia	Caused by a series of small strokes
Small vessel disease-related dementia (also known as sub-cortical vascular dementia; or in severe cases, Binswanger's disease).	This form of the disease is manifested by damage being caused to the tiny blood vessels that are located deep inside the brain.

There are other conditions that can also cause damage to the brain's vascular system. These include conditions such as: high blood pressure; high cholesterol; diabetes; heart problems.

Pick's Disease/ Frontotemporal dementia

Frontotemporal dementia is a lesser known, and far less well understood, form of dementia than vascular dementia or Alzheimer's disease. The much greater salience in the public eye of Alzheimer's disease, and concomitant symptoms, has created an environment where the very different symptoms of frontotemporal dementia are much more likely to be misunderstood or indeed, dismissed.

Frontotemporal dementia is also more likely to affect younger people, between the ages of 40 and 45. This tends to compound the risk of misdiagnosis as a psychiatric or behavioural problem. As with other forms of dementia, however, frontotemporal dementia is progressive, and will worsen over a number of years, ultimately leading to the person requiring 24/7 care.

In fact, frontotemporal dementia is an umbrella term for a range of disorders that affect the frontal and temporal lobe areas of the brain. The condition is rarer than other forms of dementia, but the experience of those affected no less gruelling.

The frontal and temporal lobes in the brain, are primarily associated with personality, behaviour and language. Frontotemporal dementia manifests itself in the form of deterioration in these areas of the brain at the early stages of the disease. Symptoms of the condition will vary from individual to individual, based on which particular areas of the brain are affected.

Overall, there are commonalities in the symptoms expressed, which can be grouped in terms of behavioural changes, speech and language problems and movement disorders.

The following table looks at the symptoms within these groupings in more detail:

TABLE 4 SYMPTOMS OF FRONTOTEMPORAL DEMENTIA

Behavioural Changes	- **Lack of 'social filter'**, to help the person recognise what is socially appropriate or inappropriate - **Apathy**: lack of interest or motivation - **Disinhibited behaviour**: inappropriate language or behaviour - **Lack of awareness or insight** into thinking or behavioural changes - **Lack of empathy** and social interpersonal skills
Speech and language problems	There are different subtypes of frontotemporal dementia, which are characterised by a more marked impairment of speech and language abilities. **Primary progressive aphasia:** progressive and increasing difficulty in using and understanding written and spoken language: e.g. difficulty finding the right word, or finding the name for certain objects. There are two types of primary progressive aphasia: - **Semantic dementia/ aka 'semantic variant primary progressive aphasia'**: characterised by difficulty in naming objects, and may use a general term, such as 'it' to replace a specific word; may also lose insight into meaning of certain words. - **Progressive agrammatic (non-fluent) aphasia:** characterised by non-fluent and hesitant speech; telegraphic speech; misuse of pronouns and abnormalities in sentence construction.
Movement disorders	Less common subtypes of frontotemporal dementia are manifested by deterioration in movement abilities, with some similarities to Parkinson's disease. Signs and symptoms can include: - Tremor

	- Rigidity
	- Muscle spasms
	- Poor coordination
	- Difficulty swallowing
	- Muscle weakness

Causes

Often the underlying cause of frontotemporal dementia is unknown. More than half of people with the condition, will have no family history of dementia.

There are two subtypes of frontotemporal lobar degeneration: one is characterised by the accumulation in the brain of a protein called tau; the other involves a protein called TDP-43.

There is no cure for this disease, or any way of slowing the progress of the condition. Moreover, medication that may help to allay the symptoms of Alzheimer's disease, are ineffective for people with frontotemporal dementia, as it can intensify symptoms of aggression.

On average, people live for approximately 5-7 years after diagnosis.

Dementia with Lewy Bodies

Lewy bodies were first identified by Frederick Lewy in 1912. They are small, round pieces of protein that develop in brain cells. They disrupt normal processes in the brain and can cause dementia.

Symptoms of dementia with Lewy bodies

- Some symptoms are similar to Alzheimer's and Parkinson's disease: slowness; trembling limbs; muscles stiffness; voice changes in tone or volume.
- Other unique symptoms
    - **Hallucinations:** sometimes can be very detailed, featuring people or animals.
    - **Disturbed sleep:** especially at night, involving nightmares and hallucinations.

- **Variations in abilities:** throughout day/ or hour by hour.
  - Onset: usually after the age of 65.

Treatment

There is no cure for Dementia with Lewy Bodies, as with Alzheimer's Disease.

Similar drugs as used for Alzheimer's and Parkinson's are used for helping to control the symptoms of this form of dementia.

Nevertheless, drugs for Parkinson's can sometimes aggravate confusion and hallucinations, despite improving physical symptoms.

Neuroleptics: these are powerful tranquilising drugs used for people with serious mental illness. They can cause serious side-effects for people with Lewy bodies. If these are prescribed, individuals will need to be monitored very closely.

Creutzfeldt Jakob Disease (CJD)

This form of dementia is very rare, and much more aggressive and faster in its progression. It leads to rapid death of brain cells, and spongiosis.

It is possible to be infected for many years without any symptoms. Once symptoms appear, however, the disease can progress frighteningly rapidly, to the extent that the patient may potentially die even with six months of diagnosis.

The symptoms of this devastating condition are as follows:

- Initially: lapses in memory; mood swings; apathy
- And then gradually: increasing clumsiness; unsteadiness; slurred speech.
- In the final stages: Lack of control over body; inability to move or speak.

Different Types of CJD

Sporadic CJD	Most likely to affect people over the age of 50.
Familial CJD	Has a genetic cause. Usually affects people between the ages of 20 and 60, and lasts longer than other types of CJD. After diagnosis, people live between 2-10 years.
Iatrogenic CJD	Disease is passed from contact with infected body tissue. Surgical instruments used on people with CJD are disposed of, because sterilisation does not kill the infection.
Variant CJD	First recognised in 1996, called 'Mad Cow Disease'. Caused by beef products contaminated with spongiform encephalopathy (BSE). Usually affects younger people. No known cure or treatment.

Huntingdon's Disease

Huntingdon's Disease is a hereditary disease. It is present from birth, although the symptoms do not tend to appear until the person has reached their mid-thirties or early forties. The condition is progressive, and there is no cure.

There are drugs that are able to help manage some symptoms such as depression, mood swings and also physical symptoms such as involuntary movements.

Symptoms

- Deterioration in parts of brain responsible for planning/ organising
- Difficulty doing everyday tasks, like washing dishes.
- People become rigid in behaviour and very dependent on routines.
- May become disinhibited: e.g. make inappropriate sexual advances.
- Become less concerned about personal hygiene.
- Lack sympathy and empathy. May appear cold and uncaring.

- Short-term memory loss.
- Irritability/ sudden uncontrollable bouts of anger.
- Unlike Alzheimer's, individuals do not lose recognition of people or places, or understanding of what is happening around them.

Dementia Syndrome or 'Mixed Dementia'

'Mixed dementia' is the term applied, where a person has more than one diagnosable type of dementia. There are different combinations possible, although most common is a combination of Alzheimer's disease and vascular dementia. It is also possible to have, for example, Alzheimer's disease as well as Dementia with Lewy Bodies.

Having more than one coexisting form of dementia, affects approximately 10% of people with dementia, and is also more common amongst those over the age of 75.

The term 'dementia syndrome' describes the manifestation of a group of related symptoms, that may derive from one or more subtypes of dementia, and which together exacerbate the ongoing decline of brain functioning.

HIV-Associated Dementia

HIV is a virus (also known as human immunodeficiency virus) that can cause system-wide infection, which weakens the individual's immune system. This can make the person more susceptible to other infections or diseases, however effects on cognitive functioning affect nearly 50% of people with HIV. This condition is known as HIV-associated neurocognitive disorder (HAND):

Symptoms:

- Difficulties with short-term memory
- Learning
- Slowness of thinking
- Concentration difficulties
- Difficulties with decision impairment

- Physical unsteadiness
- Mood changes
- Problems with sense of smell

Treatment:

Antiretroviral drugs can help to prevent cognitive impairments getting worse, and can sometimes reverse the cognitive damage already caused by HIV.

STATISTICS

There is a persistent challenge in trying to obtain accurate statistics reflecting the number of people with dementia in the UK. This is because dementia in its early stages, tends to display very subtle symptoms that are often very similar to other conditions, and is therefore difficult to diagnose. The condition is very gradual in progression, and therefore an individual may have been living with a worsening condition for a long time before receiving a diagnosis. Furthermore, there are many individuals who may be affected by the primary diagnosis of another condition, such as a severe mental health condition, physical or learning disability. Certain conditions increase the risk of developing dementia in coexistence with other pre-existing symptoms, and yet they also often struggle to obtain the dementia diagnosis.

The current number of people with a diagnosis of dementia in the UK is 537,097, at the present time of writing[ii]. For reasons mentioned above, however, this is in large part a significant underestimate. In fact, the estimated total for the actual number of people living in the UK with dementia, is thought to be about 850,000[iii].

Shift one's glance from the present day to the future, and one can quickly see that the problem, already large, is only set to get worse. It has been estimated, that by 2025, the number of people in the UK with dementia will increase to approximately 1 million. And by 2050, this figure will increase to two million[iv].

The cost of dementia can be seen in both economic and societal terms. One estimate puts the current cost of dementia in the UK at £26 billion[v]. The majority of dementia costs are due to informal care at £11.6 billion (44.2%), with social care costing £10.3 billion (39.0%) and healthcare costs £4.3 billion (16.4%).

The number of informal carers in the UK looking after people with dementia, is approximately 700,000. Whether out of a sense of duty, devotion or desperation, family carers take on huge caring responsibilities for their loved ones. They often do not want any 'reward' or 'recognition', because their motivation is love. On the other hand, many carers also have an imperative to receive some sort of financial or social support, to meet their own basic needs, let alone those of the person they are looking after. What is undoubtedly true, nonetheless, is that without the tireless efforts of such people, the state would find itself having to discharge the caring responsibility itself. The savings that family carers afford the state, has been estimated to be approximately £6 billion.

Hospitals can be extremely frightening places for people with dementia. Managing at home can be a challenge in itself, when one is losing one's short term memory, feeling disorientated, and communicating is becoming an ever-increasing challenge. Imagine having those problems compounded by being in an unfamiliar place, surrounded by unfamiliar people, while being unwell – and no doubt, feeling frightened as well. People with dementia in hospitals often experience delayed discharge, as health practitioners try to grapple with the problem of not having enough alternative care settings that would be safe enough to discharge dementia patients to.

It has been estimated that approximately one quarter of hospital beds are occupied by people living with dementia who are over 65 years of age[vi]. The number of people living with dementia who will need palliative care by 2040 in England and Wales, is expected to quadruple[vii].

Furthermore, with life expectancy increasing, and the quality of medical interventions able to maintain life improving year on year, it is also to be expected that the complexity of conditions affecting people with dementia is also set to increase. It is currently estimated that 72% of people living with dementia also have another medical condition or disability. This further has an influence on cost, in terms of costs for medication, care and support[viii].

These are formidable problems to address by decision-/ and policy-makers at all levels of government and society. At the centre of all it, are not just 'individuals': but wives and husbands, mothers and fathers, grandparents, friends, neighbours, and even more vulnerable people in mental health hospitals, prisons or homeless shelters. These are problems that require concerted and sustained effort, on a huge scale, to address.

TABLE 5 SUMMARY OF STATISTICS RELATING TO DEMENTIA

- At the time of writing, there are 537,097 diagnosed with dementia in the UK.
- The actual number of people living with dementia in the UK, is estimated to be 850,000.
- One million people in the UK will have dementia by 2025. This will increase to two million by 2050.
- The current cost of dementia in the UK is £26 billion.
- There are 700,000 informal carers for people living with dementia in the UK.
- In England and Wales, the number of people living with dementia who need palliative care will almost quadruple by 2040.
- ¼ of hospital beds are occupied by people with dementia who are over 65.
- 72% of people living with dementia also have another medical condition or disability.

PREVALENCE OF DIFFERENT TYPES OF DEMENTIA

TABLE 6 RATES OF DIAGNOSIS OF DIFFERENT TYPES OF DEMENTIA[ix]

Alzheimer's disease	2/3rds of cases of dementia are attributed to Alzheimer's disease, which represents approximately 500,000 people in the UK
Vascular dementia	1:5 or 20% of people are diagnosed with vascular dementia, which is therefore the second most common cause of dementia.
Dementia with Lewy bodies	15% of people with dementia are diagnosed with dementia with Lewy bodies (DLB).
Frontotemporal dementia	Approximately 5% of people are diagnosed with frontotemporal dementia (FTD).
Early-onset Dementia	About 4% of people with Alzheimer's disease are under the age of 65, representing more than 42,000 people.

POTENTIAL FACTORS THAT CONTRIBUTE TO THE DEVELOPMENT OF DEMENTIA – RISK FACTORS

Risk factors are just that: they are factors that increase the 'risk' of developing a disease. But they are not the same as 'causes'. We will look at an array of risk factors towards developing dementia later in life in this coming section. It is important, however, not to relinquish awareness or commitment to maintaining a healthy lifestyle, which is often more significant than the risk factors themselves.[x]

GENETICS

In general, it is thought that if there is a family history of Alzheimer's disease, then this can transmit a slightly increased risk to later generations within that family.

Certain types of dementia have a stronger genetic link than others. For example, it is thought that there is a strong genetic link behind Huntingdon's disease. Scientists have also discovered some genes that appear to increase the risk of developing Alzheimer's disease, such as one which is called apolipoprotein E.

Nonetheless, as mentioned above, many people never do go on to develop Alzheimer's disease, even if they do have a family history of it.

MEDICAL HISTORY

The risk of developing dementia is increased if a person is affected by certain other long-term underlying conditions or diseases: for example, multiple sclerosis; HIV; Down's syndrome; Huntingdon's disease.

Conditions that compromise or put pressure on a person's blood pressure or vascular system, can also increase the risk of developing dementia: such as, cardiovascular problems; high blood pressure problems; stoke; diabetes; obesity.

In addition, conditions affecting the brain can also lead to an increased risk: such as, severe head injuries; progressive or severe mental health illnesses like schizophrenia.

LIFESTYLE CHOICES

How people maintain their everyday health, through food or exercise, can influence the risk of developing conditions mentioned above that can affect the heart, vascular system or mental health.

These are aspects of life that people have an element of greater choice over: diet; smoking; excessive drinking of alcohol; taking regular exercise; keeping mentally stimulated.

Where people do not manage their everyday lives to be healthy, then this can also potentially lead to an increased risk of dementia.

HOW DEMENTIA IS RECOGNISED AND OTHER CONDITIONS MIGHT BE MISTAKEN FOR IT

Diagnostic Process

There are a number of ways how a person might receive the initial assessment for dementia. The majority of people will sense a problem themselves and will visit the GP to try to identify the underlying cause.

Sometimes the assessment takes place in hospital. If a person over the age of 75 is admitted to hospital, they should be assessed for confusion or memory problems.

At the other times, GPs need to work proactively to assess patients at increased risk of developing dementia: such as patients with Parkinson's disease; those over the age of 60 with diabetes, cardiovascular disease or stroke.

The process for diagnosing dementia involves a number of different tests and assessments. Clinicians will be keen to avoid diagnosing someone with dementia in error, when in fact there is a different underlying illness, which thereby does not get adequately treated itself.

The GP will first take a history of the person and gather relevant information from the person's medical history. The GP will then conduct physical examinations, including blood and urine samples to rule out other potential conditions.

It is uncommon for a GP to feel able to make a diagnosis at the initial visit. More usually, a diagnosis is made when the condition becomes more advanced. In some circumstances, the GP may decide to refer the person for further assessment, such as by: a memory assessment service, memory clinic, or the community mental health team.

The next stage is to refer the person to a specialist, such as a consultant. The speciality of the consultant that the patient will be referred to, will in part depend on the person's age, their symptoms and to some extent what services are available in the area where they live, for example:

- **Old age psychiatrists:** mainly specialise in older people's mental health.
- **General adult psychiatrists:** specialise in a broader range of mental health conditions, including younger adults.
- **Geriatricians:** specialise in all physical illnesses and disabilities that are associated with older people.
- **Neurologists:** specialise in broader range of diseases and disorders of the brain and nervous system, for both older and younger people, as well as people with rarer forms of dementia.

The specialist will conduct more comprehensive and in-depth investigations: including brain scans and mental examinations. Consultants work with a multi-disciplinary team, composing of mental health nurses, psychologists, occupational therapists, social workers and other dementia advisers.

One element of the diagnostic 'toolbox' is the Mini Mental State Examination (MMSE)[xi]. This is a commonly used, and relatively straightforward tool, and is designed to help diagnose dementia, or to assess the level of progression or severity of the disease. The MMSE test comprises of a number of simple tests and questions, which assess the person's memory, attention and language.

There are a number of factors that can distort the results a person attains from the MMSE test. For example, a person with high educational background, may display less distinctive symptoms of dementia in the early stages of the disease, and attain a high score on the MMSE test that gives a misleading portrayal of actual cognitive changes they may be experiencing. Likewise, a person with poor educational background, or a coexisting disability such as a learning disability, may attain a lower MMSE test score, which clinicians might attribute to their underlying condition. Again, subtle changes that the individual may have been displaying or experiencing, may not be picked up by this simple test alone.

Therefore, MMSE is only one element of the assessment process for dementia. It is the role of clinicians to make a delicate judgement based on the scores attained, along with other relevant information, from the patient's history, their other symptoms, a physical examination, and the results of other tests, such as brain scans.

The Importance of Ruling Out Other Conditions

Dementia is a diagnosis of exclusion: which means that other conditions need to be ruled out, before a diagnosis of dementia can be given. This is very important, because some conditions can give rise to very similar symptoms to dementia. Some of these conditions, may be treatable, transitory or a sign of another underlying disease. It is vital that a dementia diagnosis isn't arrived at with ease, because this would weaken the impulse to identify and treat other potential underlying conditions.

One commonly associates dementia with signs of confusion, memory loss, drowsiness or language problems. It may come as a surprise that many of the following conditions can also cause some of those symptoms:

- An overactive/ underactive thyroid gland
- Dehydration
- Lack of vitamin B in the diet
- Some lung or heart conditions that reduce blood and oxygen supply to the brain.
- Side-effects of some medication.
- Other mental illnesses: depression; mild cognitive impairment (MCI).

Why Early Diagnosis is Important

Given that dementia is a long-term and progressive disease, it makes sense that the earlier diagnosis the better, because this enables the person to make plans and preparations for a whole host of things.

They may want to make plans for themselves, in terms of where or by whom they would like to be cared for. They may wish to make preparations for their loved ones or family.

Moreover, once an individual has a diagnosis of dementia, a wealth of medical and social support options become available. These range from medical interventions, such as drugs that delay the progression of the disease, to other therapies such as psychological therapy or physical exercise.

It is obvious that the corollary to this, is that many who even as now live with dementia, but without a diagnosis, are not receiving the care and support that others with a diagnosis receive.

What is it like to be living with dementia without diagnosis? You may feel afraid and out of control, due to the symptoms you are experiencing, without any explanation or recognition of them. Family members and other loved ones may also feel such fear and lack of support. The person affected, may find themselves ostracised and isolated, as their changing behaviour is potentially written off as 'bad behaviour' or 'personality traits'. They may already be living with other impairments such as physical or learning disability, and find themselves trapped within a 'label', that doesn't accommodate the possibility of other aggravating coexisting conditions.

EFFECTS OF DEMENTIA ON COGNITIVE ABILITIES

DIFFERENT TYPES OF MEMORY

TABLE 7 DIFFERENT TYPES OF MEMORY

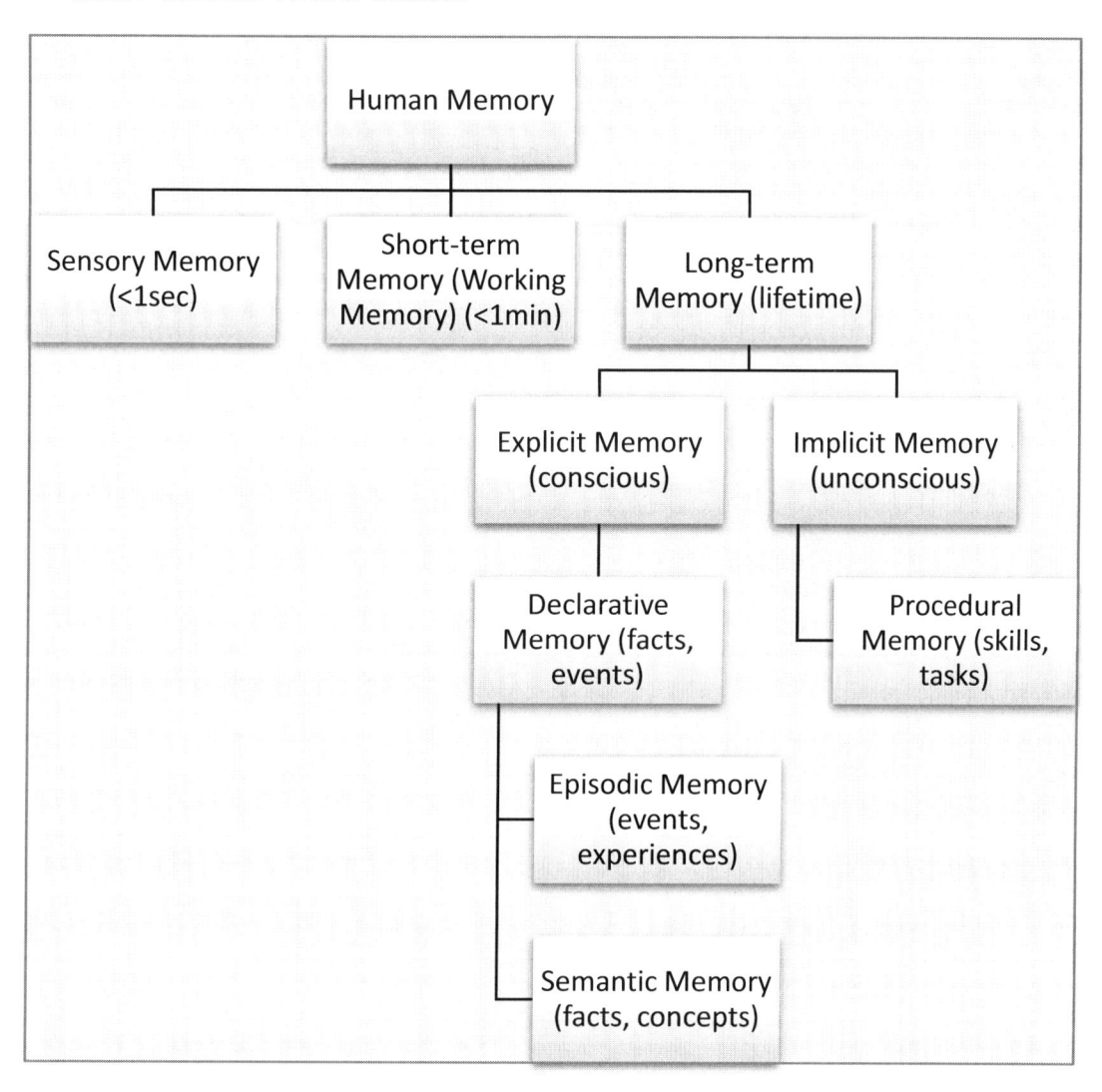

```
                        Human Memory
         ┌──────────────────┼──────────────────┐
   Sensory Memory      Short-term         Long-term
      (<1sec)       Memory (Working    Memory (lifetime)
                    Memory) (<1min)           │
                                   ┌──────────┴──────────┐
                             Explicit Memory      Implicit Memory
                              (conscious)          (unconscious)
                                    │                    │
                              Declarative           Procedural
                            Memory (facts,        Memory (skills,
                                events)               tasks)
                                    │
                         ┌──────────┤
                   Episodic Memory
                      (events,
                     experiences)
                         │
                   Semantic Memory
                   (facts, concepts)
```

People often think of 'memory' as referring to our ability to remember facts and information. In fact, there are different forms of memory, and they all work in an integrated way. Memory used to be thought of as a unitary process, but a model put forward by Richard Atkinson and Richard Shiffrin in 1968, popularly known as the *Atkinson-Shriffrin model*, debunked that theory[xii].

This model put forward memory as a process that involved a sequence of three stages, involving: sensory; short-term and long-term memory. Within the process of memory, there are different stages of memory formation: encoding; consolidation; storage and recall.

A different model, called *the levels of processing model*, was put forward by Fergus Craik and Robert Lockhart in 1972. Their model argued that the recall of memory was influenced by the depth of mental processing, which could be either shallow (perceptual) or deep (semantic), on a continuous scale. This model argued that there was no rigid distinction between short-term and long-term memory, but rather there was a difference between the levels of depth that different memories underwent in terms of mental processing.

SENSORY MEMORY

This relates to the ability to retain sensory information after the original stimuli, and relates to all of the five senses: sight, hearing, smell, tase and touch. The brain tends to retain sensory information unconsciously, but it is only processed if is likely to be useful at a later date. Usually, however, sensory memory is a very short-term memory, and lasts less than half a second.

The following are further subtypes of sensory memory:

- **Iconic memory**: the sensory memory for visual stimuli;
- **Echoic memory**: the memory for aural stimuli
- **Haptic memory**: the sensory memory for touch;
- **Smell:** smell sensations are processed in the olfactory bulb and olfactory cortex. These areas of the brain are in fact incredibly close to the hippocampus and amygdala. It is thought that this is why smells are more closely and more strongly linked to memories and emotions than other senses.

If sensory memory passes into short-term memory, this is achieved as a result of *attention*, which is a distinctive cognitive processes that involves selective concentration, while ignoring or filtering out other non-relevant stimuli.

SHORT-TERM MEMORY

Short-term memory serves as a 'temporary storing house' for information that may be needed for temporary recall, but is also being processed. Short-term memory can generally hold 7 or fewer items of information in an active state, for roughly between 10 and 60 seconds.

This type of memory is important to enable you to complete tasks. For example, when reading you need to retain the beginning of the sentence, until the whole sentence has been read and processed together. Or, when you are having a conversation with somebody, you need to remember any salient points they have said, while you wait for them to finish talking, before you reply.

Most short-term memory is not retained, unless a conscious effort is made to retain it. Retention is usually faciliated and made likely by repetition, or if it is linked and amplified by way of giving it extra meaning or associating it with some other previously acquired information. Motivation denotes a person's level of interest towards a piece of information: the higher the level of interest, the more likely it will be retained into long-term memory.

Sometimes short-term memory is described as working memory, as it is instrinsically linked to the ability to complete everyday tasks. In fact, working memory is even more complicated.

The prefrontal cortex at the front of the brain is sometimes described as the central executive part of the brain, and plays a key role in short-term and working memory. The prefrontal cortex acts as a temporary store for short-term memory, where it is held temporarily for processing, but it can also 'summon' information from other areas within the brain. The prefrontal cortex also receives information via two important neural loops: one loop transfers visual data from the visual cortex in the brain, and the 'phonological loop' transfers information from the Broca's area.

The much smaller capacity of short-term memory compared to long-term memory, can be understood from an evolutionary standpoint. When you are running away from a predator, it is important to filter out unimportant information, and to focus on important details that can facilitate rapid decision-making. Short-term memories can re-enter the short-term store, and its duration be extended, with the help of repetition or rehearsal. However, new information often quickly enters and pushes older information out (called *displacement*). Have you experienced a sense of frustration before when you are trying to count or do a calculation in your head, and somebody asks you a question about something completely different? This outside disturbance is called 'interference', and is the reason why people often feel a need to complete tasks held in the short-term memory as soon as possible, as the longer the delay the higher the likelihood of disturbance.

The process by which information held within short-term or working memory is passed into long-term memory, is a matter of controversy between experts. Some argue that there is no distinct difference between short-term and long-term memory at all. Others argue that there must be some sort of vetting or editing process by which certain information is transferred from short-term into long-term memory.

LONG-TERM MEMORY

Long-term memory serves as a storage place for information, where it is retained for a long period of time. Long-term memory encodes information for storage semantically, which relates to the way it is based on meaning and association.

Long-term memory can be subdivided into two further types: explicit (or declarative) and implicit (or procedural) memory.

- **Declarative memory**, can be described as the 'knowing what' aspect of memory. It referes to the memory of facts and events, and information that can be consciously recalled. Two further subdivisions of declarative memory, are **episodic memory** and **semantic memory**.

- **Procedural memory or implicit memory**, is essentially the 'knowing how' type of memory, and is unconscious rather than conscious. Types of procedural memory involve being able to do things like riding a bike or driving a car. These kinds of memories are acquired and sustained via repetition and practice, and are also interlinked with automatic sensorimotor behaviours.

Different types of long-term memory are not stored in the same regions in the brain. Declarative memories are encoded by the hippocampus, enorhinal cortext and perirhinal cortex (all these areas being within the medial temporal lobe of the brain), and are consolidated and stored in the temporal cortex and elswewhere. Procedural memories do not involve the hippocampus. They are encoded and stored by the cerebellum, putamen, caudate nucleus and the motor-cortex, areas involved in motor control.

Without the medial temporal lobe (which houses the hippocampus), the person would still be able to form new procedural memories (e.g. playing the piano), but would not be able to remember the events during which they happened or when they learned them.

The concept of '**priming**' also helps to bring into relief the distinctions between implicit and explicit memory. Priming is the effect whereby exposure to a particular stimulus, influences one's response to a subsequent stimulus. If a person read a list of words that included the word 'concert', and was then asked to come up with a word beginning with '-con', there would be a strong likelihood that they would say 'concert'. There have been studies conducted on people with amnesia which indicates that the process of 'priming' is controlled by a part of the brain that supports explicit memory. In other words, it is quite possible, to have an intact implicit memory, despite having a severely impaired explicit memory.

Declarative memory can be divided into episodic and semantic memory. Episodic memory relates to the memory of specific events and experiences. The emotional connections and associations with these kinds of memories are closely integrated with nature and salience of the information stored.

Semantic memory relates to the storage of facts, meanings, concepts and knowledge about the external world. Such information is less closely interrelated with personal experience, and the spatial/ temporal context in which it was acquired.

It is thought that information stored as semantic memory is derived from episodic memory, as that is the portal whereby new facts and experiences are learned. There is a gradual transition of memory from episodic to semantic memory, as emotional sensitivity linked to certain memories reduces over time.

There is a further way of subdiving long-term memory. **Retrospective memory** is where information from the past is remembered, whether that be past events, semantic, episodic, declarative, explicit or implict. **Prospective memory** refers to information that is to be remembered in the future, and is about 'remembering to remember', or remembering to perform an intended action.

These two processes are distinct from eath other, but also interrelate and are in some ways interdependent. Some aspects of retrospective memory are needed for prospective memory. Moreover, it is possible to have an impaired retrospective or prospective memory, and for the other memory type to be functioning.

DAILY LIFE WITH DEMENTIA

Relationships are the mainstay of our emotional wellbeing, and sense of personhood. And yet, the difficulties in the ability to function in everyday life that dementia brings to an individual affected by the disease, can have huge ramifications for the relationships they have with people around them.

People with dementia often struggle to maintain relationships that meant so much to them before they became diagnosed, as well as relationships that we all perhaps take for granted in our everyday lives: such as, relationships with one's neighbours, familiar figures in one's local community, friends or distant relatives.

Here, we will look at how dementia makes sustaining and creating relationships difficult as the disease progresses. At the same time, it is important to balance this viewpoint with another perspective: in that, often the obstacle to forging and maintaining relationships originates from the attitudes and behaviours of other people, and not the individual themselves.

TABLE 8 SUMMARY OF EFFECTS OF DEMENTIA ON SOCIAL FUNCTIONING

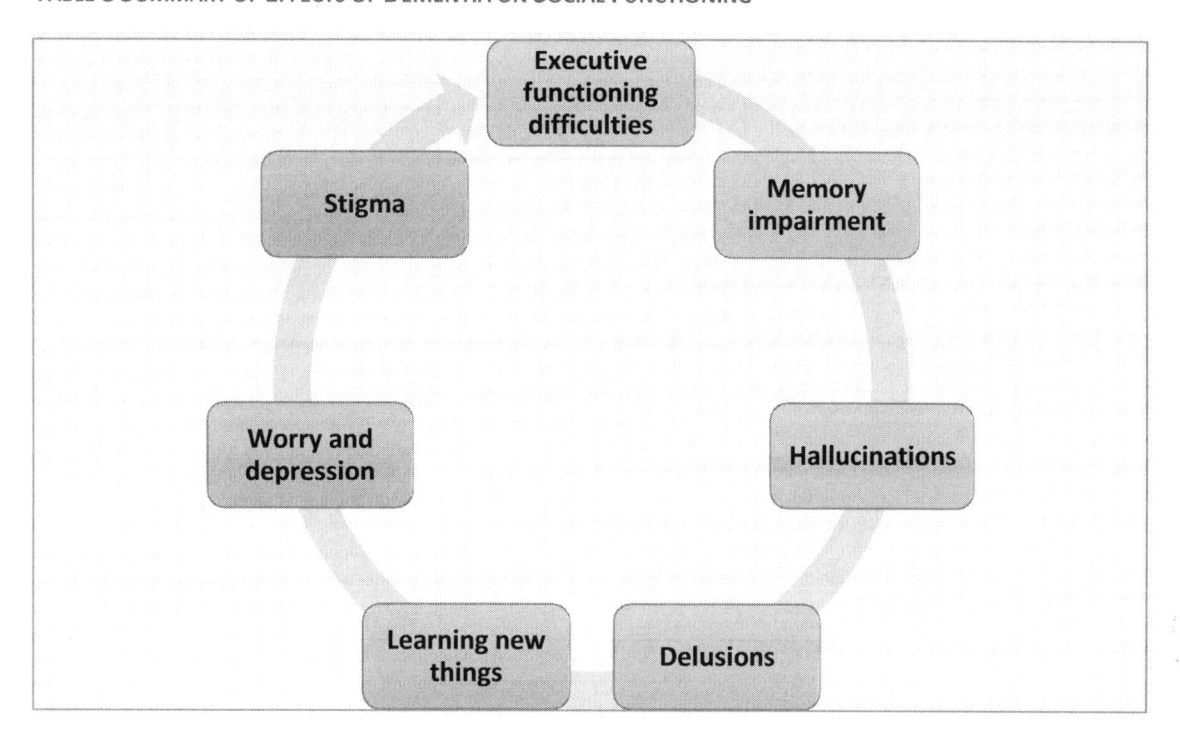

- Executive functioning difficulties
- Memory impairment
- Hallucinations
- Delusions
- Learning new things
- Worry and depression
- Stigma

In the table below, is an outline of the effects that dementia symptoms have on relationships:

TABLE 9 HOW DEMENTIA SYMPTOMS AFFECT PERSONAL RELATIONSHIPS

Executive functioning difficulties	The term 'executive functioning' relates to the cognitive ability to decide what to do next, to make plans, decide on the order that tasks need to be taken in, make decisions, or interpret social cues and modify personal behaviour.
	When this mechanism becomes damaged by dementia, the individual may display behaviours that puzzle, upset or even ostracise others around them.
	Behaviour is often understood by way of the theory known as 'operant conditioning'. This is a term that was coined by the psychologist, B.F. Skinner in 1983[xiii]. It represents the mechanisms by which behaviour is learnt and develops during childhood.

| | Behaviour that obtains a reward, tends to be reinforced and repeated. In contrast, behaviour that receives a punishment or does not incur a reward, is learnt to be avoided. An individual gradually learns and adapts to the association between particular behaviours and consequences, which then serves to reinforce that particular behaviour.

An example of this process might be where a person learns that by displaying aggressive or challenging behaviour, they receive the attention they need or crave. Sometimes this explanation is very helpful, as it helps to shed light on the underlying needs of the person displaying the problematic behaviour. Using the example above, if a person receives attention without them having to display aggressive or challenging behaviours in the first place, then the problem behaviour will become redundant and unnecessary.

The problem is that as dementia progresses, the individual may become less able to associate consequences with particular behaviours. This is especially the case with frontotemporal dementia, which leads to the person losing their sense of inhibition, understanding of social cues and an ability to modify their behaviour appropriately to suit different situations. They may become aggressive, rude and self-centred.

This is the illness speaking, and becomes less to do with 'learnt behaviours', and would require different support strategies, which we will explore later in this book. |
|---|---|
| **Memory impairment** | A common feature of dementia is the deterioration of memory, which can manifest itself in a number of different ways.

For example, the person affected may struggle to remember names, or link names to faces. They may gradually lose the ability to recognise close relatives and friends.

They may remember people from an emotional viewpoint: they may not remember the person's name, but will remember how that person made or makes them feel. However, it can be truly |

	heart-breaking for family members or friends of the person with dementia, gradually finding that they no longer remember their name, or recognise who they are.
	Often this leads to friends or family members shying away or distancing themselves from the person with dementia.
	One should strive to reduce these negative feelings and reassure others who may feel them too. This is a time when everyone needs to support each other. And remember, to reiterate the point made earlier, the person with dementia will remember how a person makes them feel, long after they have begun to struggle to remember their name.
Hallucinations/ delusions/ thought disorders	Hallucinations can come in many different forms. Auditory hallucinations can be experienced in the form of voices, sounds or music, which feel to the person as if they are coming from an external source.
	Visual hallucinations involve the person seeing things or experiencing visions, that can be simple in nature or complex. Some people may see shapes, or letters: while others may see complex scenes or people.
	People can also experience smell hallucinations. Or also somatic hallucinations, whereby they may experience a pain or sensation in the body that isn't actually there.
	It can be very hard for the person with dementia, experiencing this kind of disorder, to sustain relationships around them. There is very little general understanding or awareness about hallucinations, and people can respond in an argumentative, unsupportive or dismissive fashion.
	The key point to remember, is that if a person is experiencing a hallucination: it is real *to them*. It is better to distract and divert their attention, while validating what they believe to have seen or experienced. Getting into an argument will only increase their stress and your own.

Delusions	Delusions are characterised by unshakeable beliefs in something, that are completely disconnected from truth or reality. There are different types of delusions. Some delusions have a tentative link to reality. For example, a person might believe that someone is lying to them, or is a danger to them. Such delusions are untrue, yet they have some relatedness with 'the way things work'. Other delusions can be much more bizarre. For example, a patient I supported once used to express a belief that he had been called up to join the Russian army, and needed to start undergoing military training. Sometimes people may believe that they are being controlled by aliens. Here are some other subtypes of delusions[xiv]: - **Erotomaniac:** the person believes that someone else, often a well-known or important person, is in love with them. - **Grandiose:** the person believes they hold a position of grandeur in terms of wealth, importance or power. - **Jealous:** they believe that their partner or spouse is being unfaithful to them. - **Persecutory:** they believe that they are being spied upon, colluded against, or mistreated. - **Somatic:** they believe that they have a physical defect or medical problem. - **Mixed:** the person displays one or more of these different types of delusions.
Learning new things	People with dementia often struggle to learn new things, even though as the disease progresses, aids for physical mobility or communication become all the more important to help promote independence in everyday life.

	For example, they may struggle to learn how to use adapted telephones, or simply a new unfamiliar telephone. The person may struggle to understand or remember to keep their personal alarm near them, in case they fall or get into difficulty, much to the chagrin of family or friends. Using more modern forms of communication, such as texting or email, may be difficult for an older person (though not always: one must not generalise. Every person is different!). Equipment that is designed to help with physical mobility, such as door openers, or wheelchairs, can also be difficult for a person with dementia to learn how to use.
	With all these difficulties, it's important to try to introduce new technology or equipment early on during the disease, to give the person a better chance at getting used to it before the condition worsens. If a person struggles to learn how to use something, it is important not to blame the person, but try to think of a constructive solution.
	Such difficulties can create a strain on relationships. The more infirm a person becomes, the more important is the telephone, or technology like the mobile phone, technology, email, or personal alarms, both to keep in touch with family and loved ones, and to keep safe. It's important to empathise and make allowances for the increasing limitations a person with dementia will gradually experience.
	While it's always good to try new things, and this is usually worth doing, make sure the focus is on devising solutions that work for the person with dementia, and things that they want: not idealistic ideas that are difficult to achieve, and may be counterproductive along the way.
Worry/ depression	Receiving the diagnosis of dementia can be intensely frightening for both the person concerned, and their loved ones. The complex array of emotions will be different for each person, and will be influenced by other factors or circumstances.
	For example, if the person receiving the diagnosis is under the age of 65, the fear of the financial consequences, the sense of loss and

	societal stigma, maybe extremely intense. For all people however, the feelings will include fear, bewilderment, insecurity and a certain amount of grief for one's memories that may gradually fade away, and for how one's family and loved ones will be affected. People affected with the dementia diagnosis, often feel like they must isolate themselves, not to 'be a burden' on others, and become quite withdrawn and depressed. Every person is different, and other people might respond differently. Above all, however, it is important that friends and family, remember that if the person with dementia appears more isolative or withdrawn, this may be because they are afraid of rejection, feeling like a burden or 'insufficient' in some way. Empathising with these feelings, can help a long way with making sure you don't reinforce them by reducing contact, not talking so much, or not visiting so much, for example. When a person is going through a nightmare, they need their friends and loved ones all the more. They just may feel scared to say so.
Stigma	In the past, people may have shied away from talking about dementia, or indeed any mental illness. People of an older generation, or indeed younger generations, may have been brought up with this kind of stigma and almost 'buy into' the prejudice. If they themselves are affected by a dementia diagnosis, they may feel intensely afraid of the stigma that they may face from neighbours, or society in general. They may feel it is almost 'to be expected'. This feeling can only reinforce the other feelings of fear, shame, grief, and the perceived need to isolate oneself. Those around the person with dementia, must try to overcome these feelings about stigma. It is important to support the person to maintain their links with the community, friends and family, and to make the most of all opportunities that life brings, regardless of the underlying menace that dementia brings, and above and beyond, to reinforce the person's sense of self-worth, self-respect and personhood.

Apply and Demonstrate

The above section will, I hope, have given you lots of food for thought. To achieve the Dementia Care Certificate, you will be expected to show how you can relate your understanding to your own work practice and work experience.

You will need to describe how dementia can/ or does affect an individual's daily life.

In your description, you can include some or all of the categories of issues outlined above, or indeed you may think of issues completely unique to your own work experience, or experience of working with a particular person.

The important thing is to show how you can link your theoretical understanding, with your day to day work in a healthcare setting.

Fluctuating Symptoms and the Importance of Effective Recording

One of the confusing and frustrating aspects of dementia, is the manner in which symptoms can fluctuate from day to day, week to week, and even from one minute to the next. Sometimes this can make it difficult to see the 'whole picture', and spot trends that signify a general worsening of the dementia overall. On the other hand, it is also important to have an awareness and understanding of triggers or reasons behind spontaneous lapses in mood or aggressiveness.

Dementia can affect the ability to regulate one's mood and emotions. At one moment, a person may appear calm and composed, but at the next moment they may be in floods of tears and appear inconsolable, or displaying outbursts of aggression. Sometimes there might be a definable trigger behind such mood swings. They might be bored or anxious about something. They also might possibly have had a long-term psychiatric condition, such as anxiety or depression, which makes them even more predisposed or desensitized to potential triggers. They might have had their medication altered, which is giving rise to side-effects, or they might be experiencing pain due to an unnoticed condition, such as urinary tract infection.

Disorientation is also a common trigger for mood fluctuations. It may be that they repeatedly ask to go home, or harbour delusional thoughts, such as that they are a policeman or an important figure, and become angered when people 'tell them what to do'. Often, behavioural disturbances can come down to the way someone has spoken to them, if they were bossy, condescending or derogatory in some way.

It is impossible to build a picture, and promote a team understanding of triggers or other symptoms that need the attention of a doctor, consultant or psychologist, without effective recording. Here are some reasons, why good record keeping is so vital:

- Helps to enable symptoms or emerging changes to patterns of behaviour to be identified;
- Helps to promote coordination between the multi-disciplinary team: including occupational therapists, physiotherapists, psychologists, psychiatrists, doctors, consultants, nurses, or health care assistants.
- Reinforces accountability and professional codes of conduct.

Relevance of the Social and Medical Model of Disability

The concepts of the social and medical model of disability are described in greater depth in Chapter 5.

In essence, there are different ways at looking upon disability (or dementia), and often one's perspectives can greatly influence one's interpretation and analysis of a problem, and the solutions one thinks should be deemed necessary to address it.

The social model of disability sees that attitude and environmental context in which a disabled person lives, as often more disabling than the condition itself.

The medical model, on the other hand, focuses on the biological and physiological symptoms of a condition, and places an emphasis on search for cures or prognosis, not improving the societal and environmental factors that will influence that person's quality of life and personal outcomes.

Here are just some examples of how these different perspectives or models of disability, can result in quite different outcomes or approaches by practitioners using them when dealing with the common problems that affect people with dementia:

Area of difficulty for people with dementia:	Medical Model of Disability:	Social Model of Disability:
Executive functioning difficulties	- May regularly use restrictive interventions to deal with restless or aggressive behaviour - May have rigid timetable for mealtimes, with little flexibility towards planning the day	- May have strategies in place to help the person make decisions, to know 'what is happening next', and structured activities throughout the day to avoid or allay boredom and disorientation.
Learning new things	- May introduce equipment such as unfamiliar moving and handling equipment, alarm buzzers or telephony equipment with little	- New things will be brought in slowly, and extra support given to help explain how to use

	support to teach the person how to use it.	them, in a non-pressured non-judgemental way.
Worry/ depression	- May prescribe anti-depressants and anti-anxiety drugs to deal with depression and anxiety.	- Will provide a range of therapies such as talking therapy, reminiscence, art or animal therapy. - Will give lots of reassurance and praise, to help maintain self-confidence and independence. - Will provide structured activities to promote exercise, socialising and mental stimulation.
Some everyday difficulties:		
- **If a building has limited disabled-friendly access**	- Would not try to find a solution, but rule out the building as a possibility for going in to.	- Would ask the building proprietor about where the disabled access was, ask for a ramp to be put in place, or simply bring along a portable ramp.
- **They wish to make a phone call to their daughter, but they struggle to use the phone call that is available because their voice is faint, and the person on the receiving end struggles to hear them.**	- May interpret the problem as just 'one of those things'	- Will look for a more accessible phone: e.g. one with an amplifier so the person on the receiving end can better hear the other person, and a speaker possibly well.

> ### Apply and Demonstrate
>
> For your Dementia Care Certificate, you will need to think of your own examples how the social model and medical model might manifest itself in your work setting.
>
> The examples above may give you food for thought, or help you think of similar or different scenarios.

How Attitudes or Behaviour of Others Can Affect People with Dementia

As we saw in the earlier section, the way in which you look upon or view dementia, or disability in general, can affect the type of support one provides, or the kind of solutions one identifies to respond to problems.

If you respond to problems to do with accessing buildings or finding accessible equipment in a negative way, you could end up reducing that person's independence and quality of life even further.

The opposite approach involves finding solutions to problems, asking for advice, not taking 'no' or 'can't' as the 'end of the issue', and can bring about lots of positive effects. This approach can improve the confidence, and problem-solving skills of the healthcare practitioners and promote the inclusion of the person with dementia themselves.

Ideas or solutions found can be shared with the rest of the team, helping all-round care for that individual; and the person will value the effort that was put in on their behalf to overcome an obstacle, and may feel a positive effect to their wellbeing, self-esteem and independence.

Is Dementia a Disability?

Surprisingly, many people often wonder if dementia is a disability or not. This is possibly influenced in some measure by the idea that dementia is just an 'effect of ageing'. However, if one takes an overview of the symptoms and everyday difficulties that can affect people with dementia, that we looked at in the earlier section, then it becomes hard to see how it isn't a disability!

How do we define a disability? According to the Equality Act 2010, then you are classed as being disabled if you have a physical or mental impairment, which has either a substantial or long-term negative effect on one's ability to do every day functional activities.[xv]

'Substantial' means where the difficulty caused by the disability is not just minor or trivial. 'Long-term', means a difficulty that persists for twelve months or more.

A 'progressive condition' is a condition that keeps getting worse over time. Any person with a progressive condition, is automatically classed as disabled. Nevertheless, there are also certain conditions that automatically meet the disability definition under the Equality Act 2010: e.g. HIV infection; cancer; multiple sclerosis.

It is therefore clear that dementia fits the criteria for the definition of a disability. What also becomes clear when this is recognised, is that it is the attitudes and hazards in society and environment that are vastly more disabling, and distressing, than just the disease alone.

CHAPTER 2: THE PERSON-CENTRED APPROACH TO THE CARE AND SUPPORT OF INDIVIDUALS WITH DEMENTIA

In essence, being person-centred is about making sure the nature and way in which care is delivered, is centred on the needs, preferences and aspirations of the person themselves. It is about *not* prioritising the objectives or needs of the service provider or healthcare practitioner, time or organisational constraints, but the needs and preferences of the individuals. That is not to say that issues relating to time, restrictions of cost, organisational ways of working are 'not important', but they shouldn't come before or squeeze out the individual needs of the person with dementia themselves.

WHAT ARE PERSON-CENTRED VALUES?

There are eight core principles that underpin the notion of person-centred support, and some examples of how these can be translated into everyday work practice, are shown in the diagram below:

TABLE 10 PERSON-CENTRED VALUES

Individuality	Treating each individual as a human being, with unique characteristics and personality.
	For example: individuals with a neurological condition such as Autism Spectrum Disorder, who are extremely diverse in the manner and severity in which their autistic symptoms are expressed, should be treated as individuals, each and every one of them unique, and not subject to generalisations by default of their autism diagnosis.
	It's important not to 'compartmentalise' people, in accordance with the nature of their disability. People with disability can, and often do, experience multiple impairments. Dementia affects not only cognitive functioning, but can be influenced by or coexist with sensory (e.g. sight/ hearing) impairment.

	What this emphasises, is the importance of being aware, and to think laterally, about the holistic needs of an individual. Understanding a person's sensory issues and needs, in coexistence and in addition to their formal diagnosis, can help deliver a higher quality and more finely attuned level of care.
Rights	Human rights are enshrined by national and international statute and confer protection to individuals in all healthcare settings: including in people's own homes, as well as in residential and nursing settings. Such legally enshrined rights also apply to individuals regardless of underlying diagnosis, be that relating to physical or mental health.
Choice	Being able to make choices, is a basic human need and fundamental to wellbeing, development and autonomy. In the past, long-stay hospital institutions for people with mental and developmental disabilities were organised in such a way that residents were denied any sense of individuality by way of clothing they were compelled to wear, lack of personal space and privacy, and the organisation of routines that fitted the requirements of the organisation, regardless of whether or not they benefitted the individual. Choice is all-embracing: being able to decide what you want to eat, to wear, to think, to do. Being able to choose is fundamental to cognitive development, rehabilitation and also maintaining one's skills and abilities as one gets older, not to mention one's personal identity. Sometimes, 'too much' choice can be confusing and stressful. But dealt with sensitively, then enshrining the principle of choice can help to lay a foundation of trust and confidence between service user and healthcare practitioner.
Privacy	It is a human need to be able to enjoy privacy in terms of one's physical space, or one's living area, as well as privacy of thoughts, ideas and relationships.

	If a person is not able to enjoy privacy in any of these areas, then they effectively no longer become 'individuals' but belongings of the organisation within which they live or are dependent upon. Privacy is a human right, and should be respected by healthcare practitioners, as a vital component to building strong reciprocal relationships with those they support.
Independence	There are different ways of looking upon independence. 'Independence' can mean: the freedom to do whatever one wants; the ability to live how one wants; to live with autonomy. There can be a prevailing dynamic of change and shifting emphasis between these two ideas, when it comes to promoting independence in the context of health and social care. For example: an individual with a traumatic brain injury, who is on a programme of rehabilitation should be supported to do as much as they can independently. At the same time, healthcare practitioners need to avoid causing undue distress and upset by forcing an injured person to do things independently that they are struggling to carry out, although they mustn't dogmatically set barriers to progression either. There are times, when providing measured and proportionate assistance for individuals to carry out certain tasks, helps to give them the reassurance they desire, and the ability for them to do as much as they can themselves. One also has to encourage people to take on new tasks or new challenges at their own pace, and not in a pressured environment. Sometimes it is better to support a person in how they want to be supported, and to gradually build in ways to increase their independence and autonomy, rather than to 'disengage' or retract support abruptly. Moreover, expecting too much too soon can damage relationships, and confidence on the apart of the person being looked after.

	When one is supporting an individual with a progressive, deteriorating condition, one requires a more sensitive approach towards promoting independence, which sensitively adjusts when capabilities become increasingly constrained, and yet doesn't 'hold back' aspects of independence unduly or unjustifiably.
Dignity	The concept of 'dignity' is about the right to feel worthy of respect and value.

A sense of dignity can be derived from respect of one's physical need for privacy, during intimate episodes of personal care. It can also be supported by the behaviour of others around you, when they respect one's personal space, belongings or private information.

In a nutshell, treating someone with dignity means respecting their worth, individuality and rights, regardless of the condition they may be affected by, or the type of setting within which they are supported. |
| **Respect** | Nobody actively chooses to receive care and support, although if one or one's carer is struggling to manage on a day to day basis, then they may feel they need that care and support.

Disability or illness doesn't discriminate: people do. When supporting other people who are experiencing difficulties in their lives, it is important that the working relationship is built on equanimity and a professional attitude. |
| **Partnership** | Within a caring relationship, there is an implicit danger in that the person providing care can be felt to be more 'powerful', 'able' or 'decisive' than the person who is being supported.

A partnership relationship is one where the carer and the person receiving that care, are on an equal level. The person delivering care and support, should adjust the care support provided according to the needs, preferences and characteristics of the person receiving support. |

	Partnership working, also means a professional attitude that embraces and allows the involvement of auxiliary health and social care services (e.g. speech and language therapists; physiotherapists; social workers; advocates; local authorities.)

LINKING IDEAS TO PRACTICE

Within a healthcare setting the diversity in characteristics and manifestation of symptoms in people with dementia is always extremely wide. There will be dominant characters: people who tend to attract or receive greater attention than others. There may be more withdrawn personalities, or in contrast, some individuals who seem to 'keep getting into trouble', due to behavioural challenges or due to greater personal care needs.

Person-centred care helps to channel energies to make sure that every service user is given the attention, opportunity and compassion they need to enjoy stability and personal wellbeing.

Underpinning the concept of person-centred care, is the importance of finding out what makes people unique and special. At the same time, the experiences, relationships, achievements and struggles that inform our idea of self-identity, are not just treasured but also private. Understanding people who receive care and support, involves respecting their right to share personal stories whether, when, how and if they want to, on the basis of trust and in the expectation of confidentiality.

For the Dementia Care Certificate, you will need to be able to apply and show how you link the ideas of person-centred care to your own work practice. Here are just a few examples of nuggets of knowledge that you can find out about people you support and that can help enhance the individuality and compassionate nature of the care you provide:

TABLE 11 FINDING OUT ABOUT THE PERSON

Special nuggets of information that can help you build a rapport with service users, and help towards delivering person-centred care:	Examples:	How such information can help improve the quality of person-centred care:
Life achievements and important events	They once captained a football team; Achieved a medal in a sporting competition; Important events that affected the family: e.g. death of a parent.	Can serve as a conversation point, which could boost their self-confidence. Could help promote understanding about sensitive issues or memories that generate feelings of sadness.
People and pets	They had a special dog, which they grew up with; They had to find someone to care for a special cat, when they had to go into care, and they are worried about them.	Could lead to finding out ways to help the service user to access animal therapy within the care setting. One could help them place special photographs of their pet in their bedrooms, and talk to them about memories that are special to them about their pet.
Strengths and abilities	They used to work in a skilled trade, such as an engineer or nurse.	You could help find tasks within the care setting that they could carry out, which would help them feel a sense of self-identity and confidence. For example, they could help get involved in a gardening project.
Education and work life	They may have had a rich educational background, but perhaps their career or expectations were curtailed	You could pick topics of conversation that spark their personal interest in particular topics.

	due to family responsibilities.

Perhaps they had never been given an opportunity to develop themselves educationally, or perhaps even to go to school at all, which gave rise to a lot of psychological difficulties.

Perhaps their working life was so intense that they were unable to enjoy much time with their families. | Or you could find simple number games, that make them feel still connected with the realm of knowledge and facts. |
| **Interests and hobbies** | They may have had some particular hobbies, such as cooking or drawing.

Perhaps they had a favourite band, or a favourite genre of music.

They might follow a particular football team. | You could help suggest, or help to source some tools to help them engage in their hobbies: e.g. art equipment; music CDs. You could check in the TV guide to see when their team is playing, or help them into their favourite team's football shirt to watch an exciting match. |
| **Likes and dislikes** | They might have restricted food tastes. On the other hand, they might like to have a variety in food, and get easily bored. | Showing an interest and being able to remember about a person's food preferences, would help reassure the person that they didn't have to repeat the same thing over and over again, and that people cared enough to remember what they liked or didn't like. |
| **Values and beliefs** | Their religious faith may be very important to them. It maybe that they do not follow an organised religion, | You could help support them to go to a Church service, or arrange a Chaplain to see them particularly if they are feeling unwell or upset. |

	but that spirituality of other kinds is still important.	You could help them to get in touch with other kinds of spirituality, such as be arranging contact with a humanist.
Routines and habits	They may have had to develop routines or ways of doing things independently, which might seem unusual to the outside eye, but are important to them because of a certain disability, or because they help enable them to do certain things themselves.	You could help support them to do things in the way they prefer, especially if there is no risk to themselves or others by doing so.
Places and possessions	They might wear particular clothing, that has a special importance to them: such as a football shirt of the team they support; an army beret; or a favourite cardigan. `	Knowing important information like this, can help carers pay extra attention to items that are especially important to the person.

BEING PROACTIVE TO LINK PEOPLE WITH SOLUTIONS

Supporting people in a person-centred way is not only about understanding them, and building rapport with them, but recognising that as a carer or healthcare practitioner, you are not the only person that is important to their wellbeing! Just as important to a person's physical and mental wellbeing, is the quality, breadth and value of other relationships

These relationships may be personal or professional in nature. The relationships people have with their spouse, children, grandchildren, nieces or nephews or neighbours and friends often have an incalculable emotional resonance, even if levels or frequency of contact can often become strained and difficult when one is in a care setting. It is sometimes the case that at times some healthcare practitioners can interpret infrequent contact from family as friends as meaning that they 'don't want to come'. In fact, it is sometimes more the case that family and friends may feel a sense of guilt, shame or regret when they come to visit an ageing, frail relative.

Often all it takes to support carers, family and friends to visit more frequently, or to be more involved in the care of their loved one, is to provide a friendly supportive environment to make them feel welcome and valued. It is also important to provide and respect opportunities for private times between friends or family, and their loved ones, while also reassuring them that there is help if they need it.

Carers can go through an emotional turmoil of their own when a loved one with dementia goes into a care setting. They can often feel they want to carry on some aspect of the tasks of caring, but feel pushed out by services, or don't know how they can contribute. On the other hand, it could be that they have health concerns or conflicting commitments of their own, and are unable to carry out any practical role in terms of caring any more, but the experiences they have been through hitherto still deserve recognition, and the emotional investment they have put in, recognised and not forgotten.

There are many sources of additional support for carers, and the following table gives a summary of some of these:

TABLE 12 SOURCES OF ADVICE FOR CARERS

National Dementia Helpline	0300 222 1122
Talking Point (where you can talk with other carers in an online community)	www.alzheimers.org.uk/talkingpoint
Find out what services are available in your local area	www.alzheimers.org.uk/dementiaconnect
Carers UK	www.carersuk.org.info@carersuk.org
NHS Choices in England	www.nhs.uk/Carers-Direct/yourself/Pages/Yourownwellbeinghome.aspx
Scotland	www.careinfoscotland.co.uk/home.aspx

Professional sources of advice, that build on the strength of a multi-disciplinary team of support, are also essential to ensuring a holistic and high quality level of care. Much of that support comes from traditional areas of healthcare profession, such as:

- Social workers
- Speech and language therapists
- Dieticians
- Advocates
- Consultants
- Psychiatrists

There are also a number of organisations and websites that can provide more specialist advice, who can give advice about all sorts of issues, from accessible telephone equipment, to clothing and footwear, to schemes such as 'Talking Books', which helps people with sight impairments to access audiobooks:

- Disabled Living Foundation: https://www.dlf.org.uk/
- AbilityNet (advice and support regarding computer accessibility): https://abilitynet.org.uk
- RNIB (Royal National Institute for the Blind) [equipment often useful for both visually, partially visually impaired as well as people with physical disabilities]: https://shop.rnib.org.uk/

CHAPTER 3: UNDERSTAND THE FACTORS THAT CAN INFLUENCE COMMUNICATION AND INTERACTION WITH INDIVIDUALS WHO HAVE DEMENTIA

INTRODUCTION: RELATIONSHIPS AND COMMUNICATION

What do we mean by the word 'relationship'? According to the Oxford English Dictionary, 'relationship' means: 'The way in which two or more people or things are connected, or the state of being connected'[xvi]. In many ways, however, this definition raises more questions than it answers.

A health and social care professional supporting an elderly person with dementia, whether they work on a hospital ward, or travel from house to house, supporting people in their own homes, forge a 'relationship' with their clients, though it is one that is mainly professional in nature. Health and social care practitioners have to abide by a Code of Conduct, which highlights the importance of boundaries, maintaining professional standards, and respecting privacy and dignity.

During the exchange of verbal and non-verbal cues by a social care worker and an individual with dementia, there may not have existed any connection beforehand, and there may be no connection hitherto after the interaction has taken place. And yet, even in the brief interplay and exchange of words, body language and experience, there is a 'relationship' of sorts.

Having worked in domiciliary and residential settings for many years myself, I feel I can remember almost every interaction I have had with different clients. I don't know if those who receive care and support services, are more or less likely to remember the names and different faces of carers and professionals. Depending on the person and circumstances: some do, and some don't. However, to reiterate the point, the quality of the relationship, however circumscribed by professional codes, time and situation, is important and does matter: it can have a lasting impact and impression on everyone.

The circumstances are very different for a family carer, spouse, son, daughter or other family member looking after a loved one with dementia. In this context, there is already a relationship built upon many years of experience, living with each other, sharing the highs and lows of life and personal aspirations. In many ways, the challenge and emotional journey that family members have to go through, supporting a loved one with a diagnosis of dementia, is very much about having to accept the new dimensions of communication, and forging a slightly different kind of relationship, while not forgetting the one that was there before, and in many intangible ways still remains.

In the section that follows, we will look at a wide range of issues that can affect communication for people with dementia. We will be looking at issues that you need to be aware of and consider even 'before you speak', as well as while you speak. We will also look at ways to help a person feel engaged and valued during conversation, and how to help overcome the many barriers to communication that can exist. Not all of these ideas or suggestions might be relevant to a family member or carer, while not all will be relevant to a health and social care practitioner, depending on the setting and context where they work. All of them will be relevant in some way and at some point, however, for a person affected by dementia, during the course of their journey.

IMPROVING COMMUNICATION FOR A PERSON WITH DEMENTIA: THINGS TO CONSIDER BEFORE YOU SPEAK

In this section, we will look at different ways people communicate. This is important, because often people think of communication as just 'what they hear', or what they happen to notice. Thinking harder about what 'is' communication, makes you look more open-mindedly, and outwardly, to notice forms of communication that are not as explicit or obvious, but equally important.

We will also be looking at the range of barriers that can exist to communication, and the importance of not making assumptions about a person's ability or capability, based on information about their disability or impairment alone.

TABLE 13 COMMUNICATION: THINGS TO CONSIDER BEFORE YOU SPEAK

Different ways people communicate	As we mentioned earlier, there are 'explicit' (verbal/ outward/ noticeable) forms of communication and 'implicit' forms of communication (e.g. body language; emotional signals).
	Both these implicit and explicit forms of communication are used for different 'purposes', whether to illicit a response or obtain a result or reaction of some kind.
	Just as a rough sketch, here are some different reasons why people communicate. Some 'explicit' reasons – to: - Transfer a message - Share experiences - Debate Ideas - Convey information - Ask or answer questions
	And some 'implicit'/ or for indirect motivations – to: - Show interest - Display alertness - Express emotions - Convey empathy
	Implicit forms of communication are often just as important, if not more important than explicit forms. If a person is experiencing barriers of any kind to communication, those indirect signals can be used to help channel energies to help identify and overcome those obstacles.
	Sometimes, simply showing reciprocal empathy, interest or emotional intelligence with someone conveying those signals, can create an invaluable conduit to create or galvanise a relationship, or establish a platform for communication, in such a way that words alone simply cannot.

Barriers to communication	Unfortunately, the language one tends to fall back on when discussing 'barriers to communication', tends to lead to use of terms like 'impairment', 'disorder', 'disability' or 'obstacle'. In some cases, it is appropriate and helpful to highlight a barrier to communication. If a person with dementia, who is receiving care and support in the community or home, suddenly has to go to hospital, it can be tremendously helpful to hospital staff and the person themselves, if particular issues, or 'barriers' to communication are highlighted in advance. Nevertheless, the sheer number of staff that a person with dementia is likely to encounter on a hospital ward alone (e.g. porters; healthcare assistants; nurses; doctors; consultants) is so great, that the likelihood of consistency becomes an ever-distant holy grail. If health and social care staff, carers and medical practitioners alike, were more abreast of the range of issues that can affect communication, and were more alert and quick to identify need as appropriate, then I believe this would be a positive step. Here are some of the different barriers to communication: **Physical disability:**<ul><li>***Stroke:*** can lead to weakened mouth or facial muscles, or damage in the areas of the brain responsible for producing or understanding speech.</li><li>***Dysphasia***: is the technical term for a reduced ability or deficiency in the generation of speech, and also sometimes the comprehension of speech, often due to brain disease or damage.</li><li>***Loss of movement or difficulty with facial muscles***: this can arise as a result of other conditions, such as cerebral palsy, or multiple sclerosis.</li></ul>

Mental illness:
- ***Difficulty expressing thoughts:*** conditions like schizophrenia, dementia or other affective disorders can affect people's ability to express words or language in conventional or expected ways.
- ***'Word salad':*** Dementia is of course, a form of mental illness, but can be accompanied by other types of mental illnesses, such as depression or anxiety. Certain mental illnesses can manifest themselves in a person's speech in the form of thought disorders (e.g. the person may repeatedly assert a fixed belief or sensation, that has no basis in reality), or speech disorders. Their speech may be muddled and mixed up like a 'word salad', or the words may be pushed together like cars in a pile-up.

Learning disability:
- People with a learning disability have a greater risk of developing dementia at a younger age, and yet are also a lot less likely to have an early diagnosis, or dementia diagnosis at all. Moreover, people with learning disability may have lacked sufficient level or quality of support from services throughout their lives, and experienced reduced expectations and support to help them expand and achieve their aspirations.
- Those prejudices can carry forward, and be intensified during later life when dementia adds an extra burden.
- Much better training and guidance is needed about how to support people with a learning disability and dementia.

Communication disorder:
- Individuals with autism spectrum disorder may experience difficulties in terms of developing and sustaining social relationships, regulating and modifying certain behaviours.

Sensory impairment:
- As people age, they are more likely to develop dementia. However, as people age, they are also more

	likely to develop sensory impairments: such as, sight, hearing or other kind of sensory loss. We shall touch on this topic a little bit more shortly. **Language/ cultural background:** e.g. difficulties speaking or understanding English.

In short, before you communicate with a person with a communication difficulty, whether with dementia or otherwise, if possible, you need to make yourself aware of any relevant information about them in advance. At the same time, it's important not to make assumptions, but to observe the person, using one's eyes and ears, and make one's own judgement at the time.

Sometimes, it may be the case that a person's care plan may suggest that they have a communication difficulty, that they themselves don't recognise or indeed disagree with. It may be that they speak English with a slightly uncommon dialect or accent, and feel frustrated that people can't understand them. Or perhaps they have grown up with a learning disability, and do not identify with, or indeed reject the labels ascribed to them by others, by virtue of their impairment.

I remember once when I was supporting a gentleman who was a wheelchair user as a result of a traumatic brain injury, which affected his movement and ability to speak easily, although he could understand everything people said to him. He received a visit from a police officer, on the eve of Halloween night, who was distributing posters for residents to put up on their front doors, to discourage 'treat or treat' callers. Upon entering the living room, and seeing the gentleman I was supporting, the police officer immediately began communicating in Makaton. Somewhat perplexed, the gentleman in question asked her politely if she could just speak to him normally!

If you don't know a person, the best way to find out how they like to communicate, is to start the ball rolling and start talking with them! Or indeed ask them. I currently work on a medium secure mental health ward. My initial efforts to get to know my clients by talking with them, were often met with expletives or rude comments! A few months on, and now I can talk with all of them at ease, even those with the most profound paranoia or personality disturbance. It's all about persistence, careful observation, and gradually adjusting your communication style according to each person's personality and needs, respecting each individual as you go along.

IMPROVING COMMUNICATION FOR A PERSON WITH DEMENTIA: THINGS TO CONSIDER WHILE YOU SPEAK

When talking with a person with dementia, it's important to remember that each and every person is different. However, there are some key points to remember:

Give the person clues	If they are starting to have trouble remembering names, or putting names to faces, when you approach, say 'Hi X! It's Sarah. Would you like to go for a little walk in the garden?'
Don't talk down to them or in a condescending way	They will not appreciate it and will not want to talk with you back!
Adjust your position	So that you are at the same height: if they are sitting down, sit down next to them, kneel down or stand further away, so they don't have to arch their head up high in order to see you. An imbalance of height can convey a power differential and feel quite intimidating. Adjusting your position, helps to give out the signal that 'you are on the same level', and are willing to listen and engage in two-way conversation, not one-way.
Be considerate if the person is anxious, or paranoid	Dementia, particularly when accompanied by other underlying mental or physical health complaints, can sometimes make people feel on edge or emotionally labile.

	If they have never met you before, and you sit next to them, if they suddenly respond in a hostile way, then don't take it personally. If they want some space, or need a chance to get to know you first, just go with the flow and let them build a sense of trust on their own terms, and in their own time. If someone does not want to talk, you can't make them.
Positive body language	Appropriate use of body language can go a long way to help avoiding sudden sensations of anxiety or paranoia. If you approach a person with dementia, with a scowl on your face, talking down to them from a standing position, in a loud voice or rushed manner, then they will interpret meaning from your body language long before anything it is you have to say. Positive body language involves talking 'with your body' as well as your voice: with smiles, hand gestures, open body language (not with arms crossed!).

The following table, shows more clearly the difference between passive and *active listening:*

Passive listening	**Active listening**
You don't look at the person who is speaking, or make eye contact	You lean towards the individual when they are speaking, and make eye contact
You may feel uncomfortable or in a rush; maybe your arms are folded, or you are tapping your fingers	You show open body language, e.g. don't fold your arms, or cross your legs, display no signs of 'clock-watching' or pressure for time.
You forget what the person has said after they have finished; you interrupt the person before they have finished, and	You ask questions when the individual has finished speaking; you give enough time for the individual to finish speaking

'summarise' what you think they were going to say back to them	
You ask 'closed' questions, which just require a 'yes' or 'no' in response	You ask 'open' questions, which encourage the individual to talk more freely in response

In addition to active listening, here are also some other practical steps you can take to help encourage and improve communication:

TABLE 14 PRACTICAL STRATEGIES TO IMPROVE COMMUNICATION

Provide opportunities for communication	<ul><li>Make sure information is in an accessible format: e.g. in large print; or in audio-format.</li><li>Encourage the individual's involvement during conversation</li><li>Use open/ closed questions according to what is most appropriate for the individual</li><li>Talk about things that will interest the individual</li></ul>
Engage with the individual	<ul><li>Allow service users to express their feelings and emotions</li><li>Promote individual's self-esteem and self-image</li><li>Support them to make choices</li><li>Minimize background noise, to enable people to hear each other: e.g. turn down/ or off TV or radio.</li></ul>
Use tools to help with engaging	<ul><li>Use objects of reference – e.g. pointing to objects you are referring to in your conversation</li><li>Use photographs – e.g. to help someone recognize/ remember names of family members/ to help them know who is coming on duty</li></ul>

✿ Communication with the Senses

We have touched on the need to be aware of one's body language, positioning and style of listening to help with communication. Communication is a complicated inter-play, that involves our minds, different people and personalities, language, environmental influences and contextual factors as well as all the other senses that make us human: touch, smell, sight, hearing and taste.

We use our senses to receive and interpret information in the world around us. Our senses interrelate with our brains to help us filter out pleasant sensations from unpleasant sensations. They influence our expression of choices or decisions, in order to try and attain sensations that are pleasant, or to cope with unpleasant ones. Humans also communicate with each other via senses, touch and sound being the most obvious.

The following table looks at how an awareness or use of sensory cues, can help promote communication with a person with dementia:

TABLE 15 PROMOTING COMMUNICATION FOR PEOPLE WITH DEMENTIA BY INCREASING AWARENESS OR USE OF SENSORY CUES

Touch (/haptics)	The term, haptics, relates to any form of interaction that involves touch. It can refer to both: haptic communication, which is about the way in which people or animals use touch as a form of communication; and haptic perception, which relates to the mechanisms by which objects can be recognized through touch.
Sight	Vision is a vitally important mechanism for people to collect information about the world around them, and to feel safe and secure. As dementia progresses, the brain will strive to compensate for increasing problems with orientation and cognition, by trying to make sense of the world around them in other ways. Some have argued that the phenomenon of hallucinating, is a mechanism by which the brain tries to make sense of the world, in a context of confusion. Some people with dementia can become startled, frightened or sometimes pleasantly surprised when they see their reflection in mirrors.

	A gentleman I once supported, would often go outside to talk to his reflection in the window, who he regarded as his 'friend'. Although there were also moments when he and the reflective presence argued very vociferously. If a person with dementia becomes frightened or upset when they see their reflection in mirrors, you may want to consider moving the mirrors or limiting their use somehow. Another complication of dementia, coupled with sight impairment, is that the person – due to their cognitive decline – are unable to comprehend 'why they can't see.' One gentleman with sight and hearing impairment, would get up regularly in the night, and sometimes fall when he tried to find his bed: due to the dementia, he could no longer understand that he couldn't see, to help him differentiate between night and day. The double complication of hearing impairment makes it even harder for people. A lot of empathy, patience and sensitivity is needed for people with dementia who are also affected by sensory loss. Imagine waking up in the morning, and seeing a strange face looking down at you, and not knowing who they were. When approaching someone with sensory loss, use gentle touch, to make them aware of your presence without startling them. If you have to go, tell them where you are going, and how they can summon help if they need to know where you are. Above all, it's important to make sure that people with dementia have regular check-ups to monitor their sight and hearing, and to ensure that any tools they have to help them, like glasses or hearing aids, are regularly looked after, maintained and that they are supported to use them.
Hearing	As with sight, it is very important that people with dementia receive regular hearing assessments. Being affected by hearing loss, can increase the cognitive load on the brain, and exacerbate confusion and other dementia symptoms. If someone with dementia is affected by hearing impairment, it is important to make sure that their hearing aid is regularly maintained, and in good working order.

	You can also use other steps to help a person with hearing loss to communicate. You could write things down. You could position yourself in front of them while talking to them, so that they can lip read, which can help them reach the meaning of what you are saying, together with the snippets that they can hear.
Smell	Our sense of smell is often linked in very fundamental way with the formation and recall of memories, particularly memories formed in early childhood. When you recall a memory from childhood, you can often remember the smell that was associated with that memory as well, particularly if there is an emotional connection. There is a certain distinctive smell that I associate with my grandmother's stone cottage in Norfolk, and the musty smell of the old church organ that was in the back room that I used to sit at and pound on the keys with my little fingers. I can even just about remember the smell of my grandmother's cardigan, when I had a cuddle with her.

Smell is an interesting sense, and not often considered as much as it should be. Smell is also often subconsciously linked to mental associations to do with routine. When we smell toast, we know it is breakfast time. Many of us love the aroma of pleasant-smelling bath salts or shower gels, which make us feel fresh and 'ready for the day'.

If a person with dementia is struggling with their level of appetite to eat at meal-times, then why not prepare a casserole to bubble away for a couple of hours in the background, to create a mouth-watering aroma that slowly develops a sense of appetite and desire to eat? If time does not allow that, how about prepare some soup on the hob, or cook meals in the oven, rather than in the microwave, to create an aroma that can enervate the senses and create a sense of appetite and interest in food? I'd say this is more exciting and appealing than suddenly presenting them with a plate, composed of tastes and aromas, that the person isn't in the least prepared for or interested in. |
| **Taste** | One might wonder, what has taste got to do with communication?

However, it is one of the primary tastes that develop in babies, as they learn distinctions between objects, textures and tastes by putting things |

in their mouth, often to the chagrin of their mothers. Taste also has a complex relationship with memory and our sense of personhood as well.

In encouraging a person with dementia to eat, it is often better to stick to food that they like, and have a connection with. Rather than preparing a microwave meal, or a complicated meal with unfamiliar flavours, if someone's 'food heaven' is bean on toast, then why not! Or if the person only wants to eat their pudding, such as rice pudding or bananas, don't remove what they like.

It is more important that a person gets the calories and basic vitamins that they need to survive, rather than an ideal diet, which can be almost impossible to achieve.

Analytical Skills

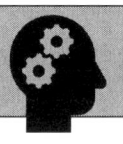

Although there was a lot discussed in the earlier section, you will find here lots of ideas and examples to help you answer some of the questions that you will encounter, as part of the Dementia Care Certificate.

Using theory to answer questions:

How would you use a person's life history to help improve communication?	- To help find out if they have any other underlying conditions: e.g. physical disability; mental illness; learning disability; communication disorder; sensory impairment; language/ cultural background.
What ways are there of finding out about the strengths and preferences, in terms of communication, of an individual with dementia?	- Use techniques of active listening rather than passive listening, to get to know the person and build up a rapport - Read the care plan, or find out information about the person from more experienced colleagues, family, friends or other healthcare professions (e.g. Speech and Language Therapist; GP) - Find ways to create more opportunities to engage in conversation: e.g. use open questions; find things of interest to the individual to talk about
Describe issues affecting communication that can arise from different kinds of factors: e.g. underlying physical condition; environmental; emotional)	- Body language, position or attitude of the person communicating with them; internal factors - e.g. paranoia/ anxiety/ delusions; background noise - Availability of tools to help with communication: e.g. objects of reference; photographs - Need to be aware of other underlying sensory impairments: e.g. sight/ hearing.

VALIDATION APPROACH VERSUS REALITY ORIENTATION

Supporting people affected by thought disorders, delusions or hallucinations, that often accompany progressing dementia symptoms, requires intuition and skill. Often healthcare practitioners respond to such issues by instinct anyway.

However, the challenges that such symptoms present can be intensified when the individual also has perseverative problems (i.e. repeats the same thought or request over and over again, despite the original trigger having gone, or a response having been given).

These complicating factors can put added pressure on healthcare practitioners, making it all the more important that they recognise and promote best practice within themselves as a team, in order to best support an individual with extremely distressing mental health issues.

A validation approach means:

- To show an empathy towards the emotional bearing and feelings of the person, that lie behind the outward expression of a thought disorder, delusion or hallucination;
- To show an interest in the content and perception of the thoughts expressed by the person with dementia;
- Not to dismiss, argue or demean the perceptions of the person being supported;
- To support the person with dynamic, creative and interpersonal ways to divert them from their perceptive disorder;
- To find holistic ways to support the person to maintain and regulate their mood and thought processes: including sensory stimulatory activities; structured routines and proactive support.

A reality orientation approach means:

- To point out the error or misconception of a person's thought processes
- Can help deliver immediate essential information needed to avert a person from a potential embarrassing or dangerous situation: e.g. they are about to cross the road without any attention to traffic; if they say unpleasant words to close family and friends, due to a mood lapse or a transitory difficulty in recognising visitors.

Deciding whether to adopt a validation or a reality orientation approach, is down to discretion, as well as quick and sensitive interpretation of situations. It's impossible to 'get it right' all the time.

However, both as an individual and as a team, it is important to develop knowledge, rapport and understanding of people with dementia who are being cared for, and to share insights to promote consistency and quality of care, particularly at times that are fraught with panic or distress.

CHAPTER 4: UNDERSTAND EQUALITY, DIVERSITY AND INCLUSION IN DEMENTIA CARE

The notions of equality and diversity are mutually dependent and interrelated. That is because the principle of equality begins with the understanding that **we are not all the same!**

Accepting and respecting the fact that we are different – be that in terms of different personalities, characteristics, needs, abilities or likes and dislikes – is essential to ensure that people are treated equally.

FIGURE 1 EQUALITY AND EQUITY

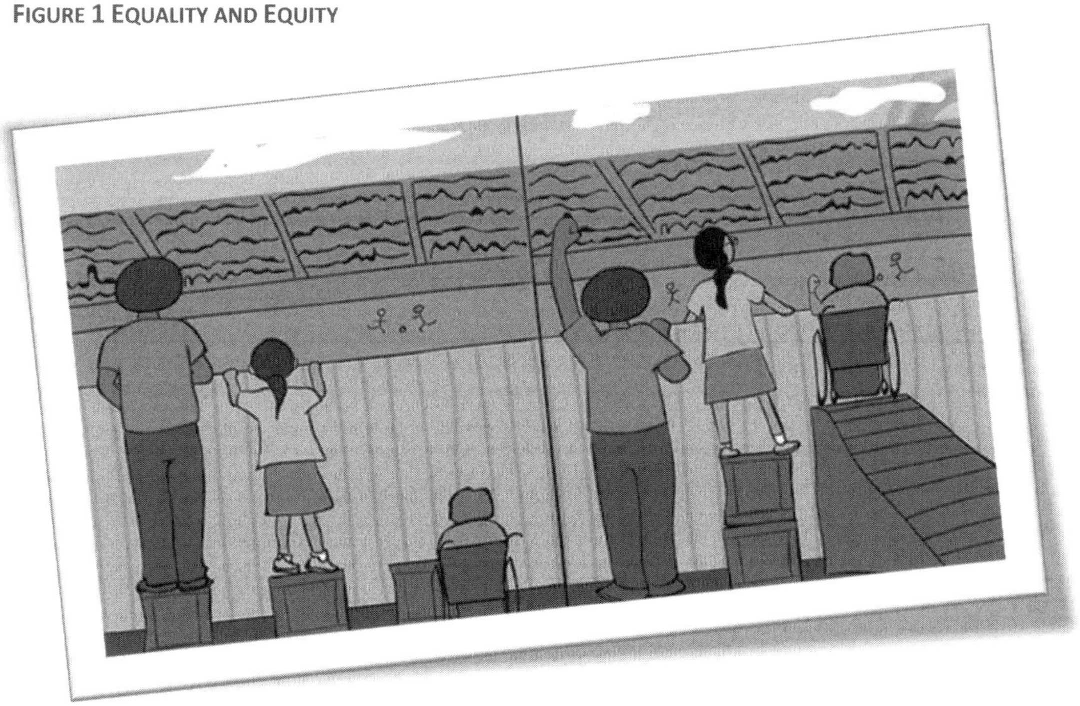

Often the relationships of family and friends with a person with dementia, can change over time after their diagnosis. Even worse, sometimes these relationships become strained or fractured before the person has had an accurate diagnosis.

It can sometimes take a little while before families, let alone the individual concerned, realises that the symptoms being manifested are due to a progressive condition.

Sometimes the symptoms exhibited can look like argumentativeness, laziness or being self-centred. If relationships with a family member beforehand were already strained, then it may be harder for initially subtle behavioural changes to be taken note of. Paradoxically, in families where there is more emotional stability and closeness, symptoms of dementia may be more quickly noticed, and yet cause greater distress earlier on as well.

Families cope in different ways with the journey of dementia. However, being aware of concepts of equality and diversity, can help make sense to a confusing and bewildering set of circumstances. Often it is the family who are craving for help, recognition or validation of their struggles as much as the person with dementia themselves.

Analytical Skills

For your Dementia Care Certificate, it is important to learn how to identify and analyse some of the different issues we have touched on in this section, in case studies.

Here is an example of a case study, and how one might analyse it:

Case Study:

Mrs P is a 78 year old lady with vascular dementia. Her family helped to arrange her a place in a residential home, when her difficulties with memory and disorientation were making her increasingly unsafe in her own home. She would regularly leave her home, and wander around town until she got lost, and talk to strangers.

In the first few months when she first came to her new home, she was extremely fearful and blamed everyone around her for what had happened to her. She was particularly withdrawn and negative when her family came to visit her, which made them upset, and their visits seemed to reduce from weekly to monthly. Mrs P began to shout out when she was upset that 'no one cared about her anymore'.

The home decided to adopt a positive behavioural support model to help ease Mrs P's anxiety and behavioural issues. Her care coordinator tried to gather as comprehensive a picture as possible about Mrs P's life history and significant life events, through talking with her herself, her neighbours, friends, family and GP.

When Mrs P began to show expressions of anger or frustration, staff would respect her personal space, and offer support when she appeared ready. Rather than ignoring her feelings, or taking things personally, staff listened, acknowledged and validated her feelings.

It was highlighted that Mrs P used to be a senior nurse. Staff therefore tried to find her little jobs to help make her feel valued, listened to, and mentally stimulated. She would accompany one of the nurses to the pharmacy to collect prescriptions etc. She enjoyed being asked her advice or to offer support for other residents at a later stage in their dementia. She was given a key to her own room, and staff helped engage her in decorating it in a way that she liked, and to help decide in where to hang the pictures.

Her mood lifted, and she became more humorous and confiding in staff. She would say she enjoyed 'working' a full shift with the day staff, before taking herself to bed when the night staff arrived.

Explore the following questions:

Why do you think Mrs P felt excluded, or blamed others around for how she was feeling?	- Struggling to get used to new things/ new environments - Needed extra reassurance - Needed others to validate her feelings and anxieties
Why was it important to find out important	- To help find out what's important to her

aspects from Mrs P's life history and to treat her as a unique individual?	- To help find meaningful activities or to talk about things which are important to her - So, she can feel like a valued individual, which will help her develop trust in the staff and her surroundings.
How could you help Mrs P's family understand her needs and preferences?	- Be supportive of when they come to visit, especially when they leave, and give them reassurance if they feel upset in any way - Encourage them to be involved in caring for their loved one if they are able to do so – e.g. go for walks together, or help during mealtimes. - Provide support or advice if they are struggling as well in any way: e.g. caring needs of their own; dealing with societal stigma.
In what ways was Mrs P encouraged to reengage in tasks of everyday living and other sorts of activities, and how did this help her?	- They found out the sort of things she enjoyed doing when she was younger and at work; they found a way for her to join in or do the things that gave her enjoyment in the past; - Encouraged her to be involved in decorating her room and making her surroundings more individual and comfortable. -
What sort of misconceptions and misunderstandings about dementia, affect the way other people can respond to Mrs P?	- People can interpret some behaviours as being selfish or ungrateful. Certain behaviours could be interpreted as argumentative or self-centred, when in fact they are ramifications of the disease.

DEFINITIONS OF EQUALITY, DIVERSITY, ANTI-DISCRIMINATORY AND ANTI-OPPRESSIVE PRACTICE

Equality	Means to be equal in terms of status, rights and opportunities.
Diversity	Everybody is uniquely different, and those characteristics of difference should be respected and valued. Without recognising the value of diversity, it is impossible to attain true equality.
Anti-Discriminatory Practice	Is about working in a way that is underpinned by the opposition to treating anyone with particular characteristics differently from others, be that on the basis of gender, disability, age, ethnic origin, skin colour, nationality, sexuality and/or religious belief.
Anti-Oppressive Practice	Oppression occurs when a person or group of people are subjected to a prolonged episode of maltreatment, abuse or authoritarian exercise of authority. It is vital that healthcare practitioners are aware of the potential signs of oppressive treatment, because as a result of their experiences and sense of entrapment, people affected may not be able to speak out about their oppression themselves without considerable support. Signs of oppression can include: - Service users appear heavily sedated - Routines within the care institution are highly regimented with little or no flexibility to cater for individual needs or preferences - Service users have poor physical health, and appear dirty, dishevelled or unkempt - There is poor communication between staff and services, and little display of compassion or empathy - There is frequent use of restrictive practices

	- There is little or no involvement of service users in giving their voice, or contributing to the care planning or running of the care setting. - There is little or no support to help people with communication, hearing or sight impairments - There may be signs of abuse or neglect Anti-oppressive practice means working in accordance with statutory and in-house safeguarding procedures, to record and report appropriately any sign of abuse, neglect or bad practice. It is also about being a good role model, and being an agent for change, by making sure that new employees, temporary staff and other colleagues also share and work towards a common purpose, which is the wellbeing and safety of vulnerable people within one's care.

Why People with Dementia Can Experience Discrimination or Oppression

It is sometimes hard to comprehend why abuse of vulnerable people with dementia occurs. However, as the media frequently lays bare, the truth is simply that it certainly does happen, and understanding the factors or reasons behind this, is critical if we are to improve the quality of care and safety for those unable to speak out on their own.

In the table below, we will look at some of the reasons why people with dementia are vulnerable to discrimination and oppression:

TABLE 16 WHY PEOPLE WITH DEMENTIA MAY EXPERIENCE DISCRIMINATION AND OPPRESSION

Denial of individuality	- They may be denied attention to their individual needs or preferences: for example, given no choice of food prepared; no support for individual requirements, such as those who are vegetarian or food allergies. - No support to create a homely comfortable environment: e.g. bedrooms with possessions; with sufficient warmth and light.

Lack of support for disability or other impairment	- There may be little or no support for difficulties, such as:
	  • Mobility impairment: e.g. lack of access to communal areas; lack of support to attend to personal needs, such as getting into bed, or washing; lack of accessible toileting facilities to enable independence when attending to personal care;
	  • Sensory impairment: lack of support to have eyes/ hearing regularly assessed; lack of support to maintain or use tools to help with sensory impairment, such as hearing aids.
	  • Equipment needed to support a person's disability or impairment, may be used to restrict their independence instead: e.g. turning off a person's hearing aid so they cannot hear or interact; providing no support for a person

	using a wheelchair to remove straps or fastenings that restrict movement.
Lack of support for healthcare needs	- Lack of support to maintain dental hygiene, resulting in mouth ulcers; oral thrush; malnutrition. - There is a build-up of prescribed medication; no support to make sure prescribed medication is administered in a timely fashion; - Lack of support or attention provided to maintaining skin hygiene and skin integrity: regular occurrence of pressure sores; hospitalisation as result of cellulitis or other skin infections; little or no administration of topical moisturising creams to areas of skin vulnerable to pressure sores.
Discriminatory treatment based on ethnicity, gender, religion, sexuality or other protected characteristic:	- Confidentiality regarding personal and sensitive information of service users, not respected or protected; - Service users not able to express or exercise cultural or religious preferences: e.g. to practice their religion; to observe traditional religious events in the calendar; to be able to choose or enjoy food choices that reflect their heritage or cultural origin.
Age discrimination	- Derogatory or insulting language is used to refer to elderly people with dementia: e.g. 'coffin dodgers' or 'window lickers'. - Little or no assistance for service users to maximise their independence: e.g. by walking in the fresh air; doing stimulating activities.
Oppressive practices	- Authoritarian style of management, with little or no opportunity for service users to have voice heard, or to communicate concerns or complaints. - Overuse of antipsychotics or sedatives - Inappropriate or overuse of restrictive practices

	- Derogatory, unpleasant or uncaring language or attitude displayed by care staff. - Poor level of compliance to health and safety guidelines; frequent occurrence of avoidable falls, infections or accidents.

How to Challenge Discriminatory and Oppressive Practice

Challenging these phenomena means being actively aware and energetic about raising standards of care, preventing or reducing poor and abusive practice. Here are some important elements to the pursuit of these goals:

FIGURE 2 CHALLENGING DISCRIMINATION AND OPPRESSION

Be an agent for change, and not a passive spectator

- Make sure you are up-to-date with safeguarding training, and utilise appropriate procedures for recording and reporting abusive or bad practice.

Promote positive communication and rapport with service users

- Find ways to help people overcome communication barriers; always respect confidentiality and build a relationship of trust; reassure servcie users that they can express concerns or worries at any time.
- Work in partnership with carers, friends and family of service users, to promote social networks and support mechanims.

Be passionate about standards and role-model them

- Contribute to creating a culture of continuous improvement; be open-minded to ideas; don't be resistant to constructive criticism;
- Be a supportive team member; do not tolerate racism, sexism or other forms of discrimination;
- Contribute to induction and supporting new employees and temporary staff, to help ensure consistent quality of care and high standards.

HOW DEMENTIA AFFECTS DIFFERENT TYPES OF PEOPLE

YOUNGER PEOPLE WITH DEMENTIA

Early-onset dementia is where the condition is diagnosed when the individual is under the age of 65 years old. A younger person diagnosed with dementia, may well have very different needs, compared to that of a very elderly person.

Physically, a younger person is likely to be more physically active, and will require greater physical exercise and a more physical lifestyle to support their sense of well-being. Or course, this can also be relevant to people older than 65, but the likelihood is that this issue is particularly pertinent to people with early-onset dementia.

In terms of social needs, they may still have financial commitments. It is very possible that they will still be in employment, with work responsibilities. They may still have a mortgage that they need to pay off. They may have children or a spouse they are supporting, or may also be looking after their own elderly parents or other family members.

A diagnosis of dementia for such a person, can be profoundly terrifying. The support interventions often provided to elderly people with dementia, may fall short of alleviating the additional pressures and fears experienced by a younger person with dementia.

On the other hand, the support mechanisms that are typically in place for an elderly person with dementia, may not be as easily accessible for a younger person. They may be signposted to support from a neurologist as opposed to specific dementia services. They may need extra encouragement or support to access services, such as from a memory clinic, or community groups such as 'Singing for the Brain', which they may perceive as being only for an 'older' person.

PEOPLE FROM ETHNIC MINORITY COMMUNITIES

As the composition of the population has become increasingly diverse over the last few decades, it is fairly unsurprising that more people from ethnic minority groups in the population, are also experiencing the ramifications of a dementia diagnosis, and the burdens that it brings.

Much of the increase in the prevalence of dementia in this part of the population, is underestimated because some people of ethnic minority cultures have a stronger cultural affinity with looking after their own family members during their old age, and may associate dementia as an inevitable consequence of old age, and not therefore seek out a diagnosis.

There are further barriers to people from BME communities in seeking diagnosis and access to mainstream services for people with dementia. A particularly pertinent barrier is language. A language barrier can hinder access to information, create a sense of social isolation, or give rise to misunderstanding. For example, it has been argued that some from BME communities associate the notion 'independent living' schemes, as 'enforced isolation' that endorse family estrangement from their loved ones at their time of need which is also culturally anathema, and not a supportive mechanism that promotes independence whilst also maintaining bridges to social and family networks.

People from ethnic minorities may need more proactive support to be able to obtain accessible or suitably translated information, and also reassurance that they are entitled to and can access mainstream services just like everyone else.

The very experience of dementia can also give rise to unique challenges for people from BME communities. Whether it is an individual who has settled in Britain in the last ten years, or the last sixty years, the effect of dementia tends to render any secondary language learnt by the person redundant. In other words, such people often revert back to their original language. This can cause untold frustration and difficulties for them and care providers, and requires sensitive support and intuitive adaptation of communication techniques, such as use of pictorial methods of communication.

There is a controversy around the debate as to whether people from ethnic minority communities have a particular preference to receive care and support from carers or healthcare practitioners of the same religious or cultural identity. Some community representatives argue that this should not be assumed to be the case, and that indeed very often individuals may well prefer to experience access to services that provide a more diverse workforce. At the same time, the opposite may be true.

In short, people who may be swept under the rather generalised heading as of being from the 'BME-community', are in fact *individuals*, just as everyone else. 'BME-communities' are not homogenous, and it would be foolish to assume so, even though it is an assumption commonly made.

No matter what one's heritage, differences of education, age, location, personality and other factors, can intersect in very different and personal ways with one's nationality, family, religion or culture. Don't assume! We **are all** individuals.

People with Learning or Physical Disabilities

People with learning disabilities have an increased risk of developing dementia at a younger age. Unfortunately, their additional needs are often not noticed or recognised, and grouped alongside the other difficulties they manifest as a result of their learning disability.

However, people with learning disabilities already experience a difficulty in processing information and communicating their needs. Therefore, the development of dementia can have a profoundly greater impact on them, compared to people who were functioning at a higher level beforehand.

People with learning disabilities can benefit hugely from an early proactive effort to build in alternative or augmentative communication methods to support them, as well as medication to slow down the progression of the disease, just as it benefits people without the additional burden of learning disability.

People with physical disabilities may experience impairments with mobility or circulation. It is known that high blood pressure, high levels of cholesterol, obesity or hypertension can increase the risks of developing dementia. Consequently, it would appear proportionate to support people with physical disabilities to manage these risk factors as well as possible. Where they are not well managed, it is also important to be aware of the indirect effect on cognitive function. However, as with other people with an underlying condition, people often find themselves tagged with a 'label', and do not receive the support that others do, to address the potential development of an additional coexisting condition along with dementia.

EXTENDED READING: OTHER MARGINALISED GROUPS AFFECTED BY DEMENTIA

PEOPLE WITH MENTAL HEALTH CONDITIONS

A study was conducted by Zilkens et al in 2014, to investigate the role of severe psychiatric disorders experienced by people during mid-life, and whether this increased the risk of developing dementia later in life[xvii].

The study was based on data collated from Western Australian state-wide death records. The data was examined to detect any correlation between incidences of dementia between 2000 and 2009, in individuals aged 65 to 84, and where there was diagnostic evidence of underlying psychiatric risk factors present for at least 10 years prior to the onset of dementia. The study concluded, that there was indeed evidence that psychiatric conditions such as severe depression, anxiety disorder, bipolar disorder, schizophrenia and alcoholic dependency disorder, were important risk factors for developing dementia later in life. These findings bring into relief the importance of early diagnosis and treatment, as well as effective management of severe mental health conditions.

Diagnosing dementia in people with schizophrenia, has long been problematic. Schizophrenia has been traditionally seen as distinct from 'organic' psychoses typical of dementia and delirium. The psychosis experienced by people with schizophrenia is often described as being more 'functional' in nature. In addition, there are marked differences between patients with schizophrenia, and those with dementia. Schizophrenic patients do not typically show intellectual impairments that are as prominent as those with dementia: such as disorientation, memory impairment or other forms of cognitive failure.

Nevertheless, de Vries et al argue that this is an oversimplification. Particular cognitive impairments, such as executive functioning deficits, are in fact prominent. Attempts to put such symptoms down to poor motivation, attention or cooperation, are not credible. Furthermore, brain CT scans commonly fail to demonstrate any more than minor abnormalities, although use of functional as opposed to structural imaging, often reveal evidence of frontal or temporal hypoperfusion (meaning reduced blood flow), especially via scanning techniques such as SPECT (single-photon emission computerized tomography). SPECT is a type of nuclear imaging test, which uses a radioactive substance and specialised camera equipment, to produce 3-D images. A SPECT scan can help to reveal how organs are actually working, and not just what they look like. [xviii]

The tyranny of 'labelling' and compartmentalizing people, thwarts people with severe mental illness, just as it does other people with other forms of disability, from receiving a necessary diagnosis when or if symptoms of dementia emerge and develop. Unfortunately, there is a formidable amount of resistance in place amongst healthcare professionals in certain settings, to entertain notions of the possibility of dementia symptoms, where the primary diagnosis is a mental health condition. It remains the preserve of especially proactive healthcare practitioners, friends and family, as well as the individuals themselves, to make enough noise heard to ensure recognition of their added difficulties are appreciated, appeased or acted upon.

PEOPLE FROM LGBT COMMUNITIES

The experiences lived and felt by those we put under the term 'LGBT-community', are very different in current times compared to in the past. The stigma and fear of 'coming out' would have been much more poignant in days gone by.

It is very possible that some people who present with developing dementia symptoms, have tried to keep a very personal matter intensely secret for a very long time. If they find themselves in a residential or nursing setting, surrounded by other people with dementia, the consequences can be traumatic.

Receiving visitors from friends and family, shouldn't be more problematic for a person with dementia, who has a same-sex partner, than for other people, but in reality, if they experience discriminatory attitudes, hostility or even subtle displays of disdain, this could have a huge negative impact. Same-sex partners who have a caring role for the person with dementia, can feel excluded from being shared information, or from being able to participate in the care of their loved one, that other people take for granted.

A common symptom with dementia, is to lose the ability to recognise close family and loved ones. Same-sex partners may find themselves in equally the same heart-breaking position, but less able to speak out or request emotional support.

Keeping sensitive and private information confidential is an essential part of supporting people in residential care settings. It is an expectation of people with dementia, and their carers, that those who look after them, respect their confidentiality and privacy. At the same time, however, developing that trust with patients, and their carers, can also provide them with the reassurance and confidence that they need to indeed open up and confide about issues that are important to them. Demonstrating trust, and respect for individual privacy and confidentiality, is key.

PRISONERS AND EX-OFFENDERS

I have decided to include a section about this very thorny topic, as it is rarely touched on and indeed sometimes actively ignored by many experts on dementia. This is a lot to do with contemporary social attitudes towards offenders, with a preference for longer sentences and a distinct lack of energy and commitment to the corrective underlying function of the criminal justice system.

To quote an anonymous commentator, on a social media platform: 'I'm not sure why they're provided medical assistance in the first place. By their actions they have voluntarily opted out of society in general.' Whatever your personal view on this topic, in this section we will explore some of the main issues.

Firstly, it is clear that the number of older prisoners within the criminal justice system is increasing – fast. As a group, older prisoners represent the fastest growing age group in Britain (Prison Reform Trust 2008)[xix]. In the last ten years, in England and Wales, the number of prisoners over fifty years old, has risen by 74% to nearly 10,000, and the number of those over 60 years old has increased 8-fold since 1990.

There are four main types of older prisoners or offenders:

- Those who are over the age of fifty when they were sent to prison for the first time.
- Prisoners who went to prison at a younger age, but long enough to still be in prison by the time they are fifty.
- Repeat offenders, who have returned to prison after committing several offences.
- Offenders who were given a life sentence when they were young adults, but who are now older than fifty. (Sterns et al 2008)

We also know that this age group within the prison population, have significant mental and physical health concerns. 80% of older prisoners, it has been stated by research carried out by the NHS, have a serious illness or disability, most prevalent being cardiovascular and respiratory diseases. Mental health disorders are also very prevalent amongst the older prison population, although in the case of dementia there is no standardized assessment mechanism used with any degree of frequency across the board, and therefore we have to make very broad calculated guesses as to the level of the problem.

It has been posited that more than 80% of older offenders have long-standing illness or disability and over 50% suffer from a mental disorder. 30% have a diagnosis of depression. The estimated figures for dementia within the prison population, is something between 1% and 30%. [xx]

There are particular challenges in terms of determining the actual number of instances of dementia amongst the prison population. Prison life tends to be highly regimented, and older prisoners tend to attract relatively less attention than younger, more vocal prisoners, who also tend to receive more support from what is available in terms of mental health services. Mental health issues tend to be more easily missed or ignored. Older offenders are also themselves less likely to seek attention or report changes to their mood, memory or cognitive abilities.

There is a further debate, as to what the threshold should be for determining what is an 'older prisoner'. Some have argued that prisoners from the age of 50 onwards, should be included in the analysis of older prisoners as a whole. This is because of the phenomenon of 'accelerated biological ageing.' This term was put forward by Wahidin and Aday, who argued that prisoners of the age of 50 and upwards, tend to exhibit physical and mental health profiles comparable to those in the community of at least 10 years senior. This is because offenders are more likely to have chaotic and unhealthy lifestyles prior to or as a result of their criminal activity, but also due to the experiences of being in prison.

This growing problem is important to be aware of for a number of reasons. Firstly, it is important that prisons themselves undertake more regular screenings for dementia of older prisoners. Secondly, they should ensure that more training about dementia awareness is provided to staff and prison officers. Thirdly, it is important that information about best practice, advice and recommendations are shared between agencies and organisations with specialist knowledge about dementia and mental health, and the prison service. And fourthly, it is important that low cost modifications to prison living environments are investigated, integrated into planning and running costs, and implemented. In buildings seldom designed with the needs of older prisoners in mind, low cost adaptations (e.g. grab rails) should be borne in mind to promote independence, and to minimise accidents and distress to people affected by the disease as it progresses.

In addition, however, of course it is known that some offenders will find themselves released at the end of their sentence, and could then go on to develop dementia. Or alternatively, if they develop dementia while in a prison setting, it is possible they would be transferred to a mental health institution where they would be looked after. In such situations, it is important for health and social care staff to be aware of some of the issues that can affect the ex-offender with dementia.

Many forms of dementia, especially Alzheimer's Disease, lead to a deterioration of short term and working memory. This can make carrying out everyday tasks, such as having a shower independently, or seeing to one's continence needs, increasingly difficult. However, ex-prisoners may have spent a long time in institutions where there was little concern paid to these concerns or difficulties, which may have been interpreted as learnt behavioural difficulties instead. As a result, health and social care staff may encounter ex-prisoners with dementia, doing things in a certain way which might appear strange to a third party, but are in fact coping mechanisms learnt within a setting where there was minimal support. Some practices may include urinating on the floor, because there has rarely been support to help them to the toilet which was out of reach. Or hiding things under the mattress, because there wouldn't have been anywhere else to put personal items, or because of a habit of concealing items.

Different forms of dementia can also have an effect, to a greater or lesser degree depending on the type of dementia, on executive functioning and personality.

Frontotemporal dementia (FTD), for example, leads to a deterioration in the frontal lobes of the brain, which govern our personality and decision-making. Symptoms of FTD can include repeated vocalisation, disinhibited behaviour, inappropriate language or aggressiveness. Unfortunately, an ex-offender or anyone with a troubled history, is unlikely to get the warranted attention they need if they develop symptoms of FTD, which are often explained as behavioural problems instead. This is not to say that behavioural problems cannot evince the same symptoms at times: however, where there is an actual neurological deteriorating problem, it can prove intensely difficult to get the problem recognised or diagnosed, let alone supported.

Finally, there is also the issue of confidentiality. On the one hand, it is vitally important that any criminal history or other relevant information is shared with care providers, to help ensure the safety of care staff and other residents. On the other hand, it is also important that that information is shared appropriately, and not passed to other service users or patients, family or friends. If a person has served a sentence a long time ago for a minor offence, it would not be just to share that information with other service users or patients, would could use that information to stigmatise or bully the individual. Indeed, it would be in clear breach of confidentiality legislation. Likewise, however, where the offence is more serious, while it is important to be shared the relevant information, and take proportionate risk assessments and evaluations, it is also necessary to only share the information appropriately, and in accordance with the law.

DEMENTIA CARE AT THE END OF LIFE

Paradoxically, thinking about end of life care, while it is in part about supporting the individual, friends, family and staff, to cope when a person is dying, and the bereavement journey, is also about celebrating and valuing the life of that person.

This is all the more important because the dying process, just with life itself, is not predictable. It never ceases to surprise, and relieve me, the tenaciousness of life. Every day, is a day to be treasured and to make the most out of.

Sometimes it may appear that a person is very close to dying, and yet are able to make a recovery and 'defy the odds'. On the other hand, sometimes death can come very suddenly and out of the blue. While dementia is a terminal illness, people with dementia also often find themselves battling against more than one condition, which can give rise to unforeseen infections or other minor illnesses, which can lead to sudden deterioration.

It is my view, that end of life care parallels and overlaps with the duty of care, and overarching roles and responsibilities of healthcare practitioners. At the core of this duty, is to promote the wellbeing, safety, individuality and independence of all people within one's care. If healthcare practitioners feel that they would 'not be surprised' if a service user in their care might die in the next twelve months, then added sensitivity and attentiveness towards end of life issues, and management of them, become all the more acute.

When a person is nearing the end of life, they may feel anxious or worried about talking about the topic of dying, or scared about upsetting loved ones or causing a burden. They may feel emotions such as regret or sadness, that there is 'unfinished business', family conflicts they wish they could find a resolution to, family members they crave to remain in contact with or whose care they are worried about themselves after they die, or simply want to make the most of what abilities, interests, passions or experiences of nature and companionship they have, for as long as they can.

There is also the actual experience of dying that people can often make people feel scared and frightened. It may be that they want to die in a place where they feel safe and comfortable, surrounded by familiar smells, possessions, friends and voices. It may be that they want all of these things, but don't express it or have it written down at a time when they have capacity, or the ability to communicate. By the time they are in the palliative care phase, then it is too late to make their wishes known, and they may find themselves having to experience their final days in a hospital, an unfamiliar frightening place.

This is why supporting people with dementia to make advance care plans, expressing their wishes and preferences is so important, before their mental capacity deteriorates to the point where they have insurmountable difficulty in doing so.

Another aspect to supporting people with dementia at the end of life, is to be proactive in helping them to manage the different array of other symptoms that they can experience. Some symptoms are easier to manage through preventative measures. For example, it is more effective to support a person with regular turning or encouraging exercise, keeping them as mobile and clean as possible, and applying moisturising and barrier creams as applicable and as prescribed, to avoid pressure sores developing in the first place, as opposed to trying to reverse a pressure sore.

Early detection is also key. In its early stages, a pressure area can be relatively simple to address and to cure: it becomes much harder and difficult to reverse once it becomes an open, or an infected sore.

Gastrointestinal problems are also common for people with dementia at the end of life. They may experience constipation, and may not be able to express or explain the sensations of pain. Helping to make sure a person has regular amounts of fluid, as balanced a diet as possible and support if necessary with laxatives, to prevent constipation, can help a lot to ease the confusion and discomfort.

Mental health problems are frequently manifested as well. A person my experience depression, or severe anxiety. Anti-depressants or medication for anxiety can help a person who is struggling to regulate their mood, or which is worsening as a result of underlying pain.

As a person nears the palliative stage, or final phase of the dying process, they may exhibit a sharpened reduction in their appetite. You should not force a person at this phase to eat or drink more than they want to, but to be flexible and offer what they like, as often as possible.

Supporting people with dementia during the end of life phase, requires skills and cooperation from the whole team of professions that make up multi-disciplinary teams, which include: physiotherapists; occupational therapists; dieticians; doctors and consultants; psychologists; neurologists; or other specialists.

The above is just a summary, but for more detailed guidance, the following website has a wealth of information: Gold Standards Framework – www.goldstandardsframework.org.uk .

Rights, Regulations and other Legal Protections

The following table outlines some of the key legislative protections that underpin the rights of people with dementia:

FIGURE 3 STATUTORY PROTECTION OF RIGHTS FOR PEOPLE WITH DEMENTIA

| **Mental Capacity Act 2005** | Seeks to end discrimination of people because of reduced mental capacity.

 Five key statutory principles of the Mental Capacity Act 2005:

 - A presumption of capacity: every adult is assumed to have capacity unless it is proved otherwise.

 The MCA says that a person is unable to make their own decision if they cannot do one or more of the following four things:

 • Understand information given to them
 • Retain that information long enough to be able to make the decision
 • Weigh up the information available to make the decision
 • Communicate their decision – this could be by talking, using sign language or even simple muscle movements such as blinking an eye or squeezing a hand.

 - Individuals should be supported to make their own decisions: all steps should be taken to help support someone |

	to take decisions - e.g. support for communication difficulties or sensory impairment; provide an advocate; or support from a close family member or carer. - Unwise decisions: people have the right to make decisions that others might regard as unwise or eccentric. - Best interests: it is important that any decision made on behalf of a person who lacks mental capacity, should be done in their best interest. - Less restrictive option: any support intervention or decision should be made in the least restrictive way, and that interferes as little as possible with a person's rights and freedoms of action.
Equality Act 2010	Protects against discrimination, in particular age discrimination that can affect both older people with dementia, as well as younger people affected by early-onset dementia. Age-related stereotypes get in the way of person-centred holistic care. The Equality Act protects a range of groups who have historically been vulnerable to discrimination. The 'protected characteristics' include: age; disability; gender reassignment; race; religion or belief; sex; sexual orientation; marriage and civil partnership and pregnancy and maternity.'
Human Rights Act 1998	Protects people with dementia, who might be at risk of mistreatment and abuse, in the community care homes or hospitals. Abuse can take many forms, include: psychological, financial, emotional, sexual or physical abuse. It includes the inappropriate prescription of anti-psychotics.
Health and Social Care Act 2008 (Regulated Activities) Regulations 2014 & Care Quality Commission	Tightened regulatory and inspection procedures for health and social care providers, with aim to make sweeping improvements to quality of care.

(Registration) Regulations 2009	
Advance Statements	An advance statement is a document that states in written form what a person's wishes, beliefs, preferences and personal values are in regards to their future care and support. The document is created by someone when they have capacity, to give a guide to others to be able to make decisions in their best interest, when they have lost the capacity to make decisions or communicate them. Some examples of wishes or preferences someone might want to make explicit in an advance statement would include one's religious beliefs, if they would like to spend their final days at home, in a hospital or hospice, if they are vegetarian, or who they would like to look after their dog if they are no longer able to. If an advance statement is made, it is important that anybody involved in that person's care, are made aware about it. An advance statement is not legally binding, although anyone making decisions about the person's care in the future, must take it into account.
Advance Decisions	An advance decision is however legally binding, and is sometimes be referred to as a living will, or an advance decision to refuse treatment. There are strict criteria that an advance decision has to meet, for it to be considered valid and applicable. It's important to note, that advance decisions are not about enabling someone to help someone end their lives: euthanasia or assisted suicide is illegal in England. However, an advance decision can be used to refuse life-sustaining treatment: e.g. ventilation; cardiopulmonary resuscitation (CPR); or antibiotics. An advance decision of this nature, needs to be written down, signed by the person/ who has capacity at the time of signing it, and also signed by a witness.

| | Here are some links for further advice on this topic: www.nhs.uk/conditions/end-of-life-care; and www.dyingmatters.org/ |

CHAPTER 5: INTRODUCTION AWARENESS OF MODELS OF DISABILITY

MODELS OF DISABILITY

The idea that our ways of looking upon disability, can be portrayed through the lens of different 'models', helps to raise awareness about how each and every one of us has ideas that are influenced by both internal *and* external ideas – societal, cultural, religious or political.

We all like to think of ourselves as masters of our own minds and ideas. Sometimes, we are made better able to do this, by being reminded of where some of our ideas may unconsciously have been derived from.

In the following section we will look at the main principles that characterise these different models:

The Medical Model of Disability
Focuses on the medical condition that is seen as the root cause of the disability.
Views disability as a fixed, and directly related to the level of severity of the underlying impairment.
Sees a distinct contrast between disabled and non-disabled people
Assumes that disabled people, because of the 'fixed nature' of their disability are necessarily dependent on non-disabled people.

Social Model of Disability
This model sees the difficulties that affect disabled people, arise more from the attitudes and barriers they face in society, than the actual effects of the disability or illness itself. Implicit in this model, is the argument that if such barriers were removed, then people with disabilities could function as freer, more equal and more independent people in society, and would not be defined by their disability.
The model assumes three principal types of barriers in society, that get in the way of this goal:
- **Attitudinal barriers:** people with disability experience prejudice, stigma and low expectations in society, often due to the attitudes of others. Such attitudes can be displayed in aggressive forms, such as bullying or intimidation, but also in more indirect ways, such as denying people with disabilities equal opportunities as other people.
- **Environmental barriers:** the design, layout or construction of housing, transport, public spaces or buildings without the needs of disabled people in mind, can effectively lead to exclusion of disabled people from many areas of independent living.
- **Institutional barriers:** the term 'institution' can refer to both physical and inanimate aspects to an organisation, or a rules-based system or area of governance, that can have an effect on the ability of disabled people to live independently.

Psychosocial Model of Disability

This model proposes that the social model described earlier, is now outdated as it does encompass the subjective nature of disability. The model serves to bring back to the fore, the relevance of disabled peoples' actual disability and lived experience of physical, mental or sensory impairment. In addition to that however, the model also embraces the social construct of disability through structural, cultural and physical barriers in society.

Another difference of the psychosocial model is that it highlights the role of the individual, and not just healthcare providers or society as a whole, in being an agent to help overcome the restrictions of disability through their perception, beliefs, attitude and behaviour towards the disability.

POTENTIAL IMPACT OF THE PSYCHOSOCIAL MODEL OF DISABILITY ON EVERYDAY LIFE

- The model encourages service providers to include individuals in care planning and reviews.
- It encourages service provides to value, support and encourage what individuals with disabilities are able to do to support themselves: such as, deciding on the support they feel they need to help them with mobility issues; or in terms of deciding what level or kind of support they need to carry out daily activities.
- The model promotes inclusion and increases the person's control over how services are shaped and delivered, making them more person-centred and individualised.

DEVELOPMENT OF DISABILITY MODELS THROUGH TIME

It is a matter of dispute as to when the disability rights movement began. There is a great deal of disparity between different types of disability, not least communication barriers as a result of neurological impairments themselves. Therefore it was only until relatively recently, when disparate groups and individuals were able to organise more effectively, as a result of better communication systems and the political landscape itself having changed after other civil rights milestones, such as the expansion of the suffrage, the women's liberation movement and the civil rights movement for ethnic minorities.

There were a number of ostensible achievements in the field of disability rights in the 19th century:

- 1817: The American School of the Deaf was set up in Hartford, Connecticut. This was the first educational institution to use sign language, and to cater for people with disabilities.
- 1832: Introduction of Braille
- 1960s: Disability rights advocacy began to have a cross-disability focus: people with different kinds of disabilities began to come together to fight a common cause. What we currently understand as the disability rights movement, took more coherent shape in the 1960s, and was characterised by demands such as:
    - Accessibility and safety in architecture, transportation and physical environment
    - Equal opportunities in independent living
    - Equity in opportunities and access to employment, housing and education
    - Freedom from discrimination, abuse and neglect
- Independent Living Movement - emerged in the 1960s: steered by the pioneering Edward Roberts. Argued that disabled people themselves are the best experts for their needs, and they should take the initiative individually and collectively, to design and promote better solutions and organise themselves to be heart in political arenas.
- 1968: Architectural Barriers Act - made it mandatory that federally constructed buildings be made accessible to people with disabilities. The first ever federal disability rights legislation.

- 1995: Disability Discrimination Act was passed: made it unlawful in the UK to discriminate against people with disabilities, in relation to employment, the provision of goods and services, education and transport
- 2006: Equality and Human Rights Commission: Set up with responsibility for the promotion and enforcement of equality and non-discrimination laws.
- 2012: introduction of the Bedroom Tax (also known as the 'Under-occupancy penalty) in the Welfare Act 2012.

CHAPTER 6: UNDERSTAND THE ADMINISTRATION OF MEDICINES TO INDIVIDUALS WITH DEMENTIA USING A PERSON-CENTRED APPROACH

Unfortunately, there is no cure for dementia. There are a range of medications that can help slow down the progression of the disease or help some of the symptoms become easier to manage. However, they tend to have a window of opportunity, when their likelihood of having maximum beneficial effect is at its optimum, usually depending on the stage of a person's dementia. They also tend to give rise to other side-effects or are restricted in the types of dementia they are able to bring benefit to[xxi].

Such medications should never be seen as 'miracle cures' or the 'magic bullet'. They are there to help manage the symptoms of a person with a chronic and progressive disease, and should be used together with other non-drug therapeutic interventions. If used on their own, they can sometimes cause more harm than good.

MEDICATION FOR REDUCING DEMENTIA SYMPTOMS

Cholinesterase Inhibitors	
Effect	These drugs work by acting to increase the level of the chemical acetylcholine which is needed to send messages in the brain. The medication tries to prevent an enzyme called acetylcholinesterase from breaking down acetylcholine in the brain.
Brand names	Donepezil (aka Aricept); Rivastigmine (aka Exelon); Galantamine (aka Reminyl; Reminyl XL; Acumor XL; Galsya XL & Gatalin XL). (XL means a slow-release form of the drug)

Benefits:	Symptoms may improve for 6-12 months. For example: - Reduced anxiety - Improvements in motivation - Improved memory and concentration - Improvised ability to continue to carry out daily activities.
Potential side-effects:	- Loss of appetite; - Nausea - Vomiting - Diarrhoea; - Muscle cramps; - Headaches - Dizziness - Fatigue - Insomnia
Other disadvantages:	It is also not clear if such drugs are effective for other types of dementia apart from Alzheimer's. They may have quite limited effect on problem behaviours, such as agitation and aggression. Such drugs are not beneficial for individuals with vascular dementia or frontotemporal dementia.

NMDA Receptor Antagonists	
Effect	Glutamate is another chemical in the brain that helps to send messages between nerve cells. With Alzheimer's disease, glutamate is produced in excessive amounts and is destructive. Memantine protects brain cells by blocking the effects of excess glutamate.
Brand names	Memantine (aka Ebixa; Maruxa or Nemdatine)
Benefits:	- Memantine is recommended by NICE for severe Alzheimer's disease or for moderate Alzheimer's disease for people who can't take cholinesterase inhibitors due to the side-effects. - The drug helps to slow down the progression of symptoms, including disorientation. - Reduces difficulties regarding carrying out daily activities. - Can also help with symptoms such as delusions, aggression and agitation.
Potential side-effects:	- Dizziness - Headaches - Tiredness - Raised blood pressure - Constipation

Medication for other forms of dementia	
Frontotemporal dementia	Anti-depressants
Vascular dementia	Drugs are prescribed for other underlying conditions: e.g. high blood pressure; heart problems If the person has a mixture of dementia types, then certain drugs for Alzheimer's disease may also be prescribed.

ANTI-PSYCHOTICS

Anti-psychotics are also sometimes referred to as neuroleptics, or major tranquilisers. Anti-psychotics are drugs that are commonly prescribed to alleviate the symptoms of people with severe mental health conditions, such as schizophrenia. Indeed, some of the symptoms experienced by some people with dementia, can be similar to those with other mental health conditions.

For example, a person may gradually lose their ability to recognise familiar faces or surroundings. They may feel constantly restless or disorientated, or they may repeat the same question over and over again. These experiences are intensely stressful and upsetting for people with dementia, who may respond sometimes by shouting or exhibiting aggressive behaviour against what they feel is frightening them.[xxii]

.

WHAT ARE PSYCHOTIC SYMPTOMS?

Psychotic symptoms can encompass three different types of symptoms: hallucinations; delusions and thought disorders[xxiii]. They are more commonly experienced in conjunction with dementia with Lewy bodies (DLB), who may in particular often see visual forms of hallucinations.

Hallucinations

These psychotic experiences can involve all of the five senses: hearing, sight, smell, taste and touch. The person experiencing them, will be unable to differentiate between reality and the hallucination.

The following table explores the different types of hallucinations in more detail:

TABLE 17 DIFFERENT TYPES OF HALLUCINATIONS

Types of hallucination:		
Auditory	*Voices*	
	Can be single or multiple	'You're disgusting'; 'you're ugly' Two or more voices talking amongst themselves The voices are usually unpleasant and accusatory. In a minority of cases, voices can be pleasant or helpful.
	Arguing	'Don't listen to her'; 'He's useless isn't he'
	Commenting	'Isn't he stupid? Does he know anything?'
	Commanding	'Kill yourself now'; 'Run in front of that car'
	Sounds	e.g. buzzing, screeching, ringing. Sound of their thoughts being broadcast
	Music	Such as a familiar piece of music playing over and over again.
	Strange/ frightening noises	Such as scraping or banging.

Tactile/ Somatic	Senses of touch	Feeling of ants or spiders on your skin; feeling that you are being pushed down; burning sensations
Visual	'Seeing' objects or people, that are not visible to other people	Thinking that you can see someone who has died a long time ago; having an imaginary friend.
Gustatory	Having recurrent or persistent sensation of bad or strange tastes in the mouth	Feeling that you are being poisoned, or that food is tasting strange and unusual
Olfactory	Having strange perceptions of smells that are not perceived by others	Sensations such as smelling gas, or other unpleasant odours.

DELUSIONS

Delusions involve an individual experiencing unrealistic, mistaken or distorted interpretations about things that are happening around them. These delusions can evolve into fixed, almost unshakeable and irrefutable beliefs, which are based on their psychotic reality.

For example, they might think that 'cleaners are trying to steal their property, and kick up dust to try and suffocate them'. Or they might think that they are under threat by aliens or spies.

On the other hand, some delusions can be grandiose: for example, they might think that they are a prophet, or a divine figure, or that they are a member of the royal family.

Sometimes, the origin of the delusion may be a sensory trigger that has occurred in their immediate surroundings, and they have misinterpreted the sensory information. For example, they may feel hot or be having trouble breathing as a result of asthma, and this triggers a psychotic delusional thought that they are being attacked by dust.

Over time, delusions can develop extended meaning and lead to additional layers of delusions. For example, they may have a delusion that they are being watched, and this could evolve into a delusion that an alien force is controlling them.

This might also lead to a state of 'hyper-vigilance', in that they are sensitive to any sign or behaviour exhibited by others to support their distorted delusional beliefs.

Paranoid delusions are delusions that consist of the person feeling like they are being watched or persecuted.

While a person is experiencing these delusions, they are more at risk of developing aggressive or violent behaviour towards those they feel under threat by, although they are often more likely to hurt themselves than to hurt other people.

TABLE 18 DIFFERENT TYPES OF DELUSIONS

Persecutory delusions	Feeling that either you or your loved ones are being watched or persecuted.
Delusions of control	Falsely believing that your body, thoughts or feelings are being manipulated or controlled by something or someone externally (e.g. an alien; governmental force).
Thought broadcasting	Thinking that your thoughts are being stolen from you, and are being broadcast for others to be able to listen in to.
Thought insertion	Believing that thoughts are being stolen or taken by some external force or person.
Thought withdrawal	Believing that thoughts are being stolen or taken by some external force or person.
Delusions of guilt	Thinking that you are responsible for a terrible act of crime.
Somatic delusions	An unpleasant sensation that something is wrong with your body, and that it has changed somehow or is diseased.
Grandiose delusions	Believing that you are a God, or a prophet, or the King/ Queen.
Delusions of reference	According strange meaning or importance to external events, objects or activities. E.g. Believing that an argument on the television is about you.

Thought disorders

Thought disorder manifests itself when a person with severe psychosis, begins to talk in incoherent or unintelligible sentences, and invent their own words or phrases to things: e.g. 'astral projection'; 'astral plane'.

Sometimes these jumbled sentences together with word inventions, are described as 'word salad'.

Development of Anti-Psychotics: Risks and Benefits

Originally, anti-psychotic drugs were introduced primarily to treat people with severe mental health conditions that frequently gave rise to psychosis, such as schizophrenia. The first types of anti-psychotics were called 'typical' antipsychotics, or major tranquillisers. Examples include: thioridazine; haloperidol; stelazine. These are rarely prescribed now, as they can frequently cause significant side-effects, affecting motor control in particular.

In an effort to overcome the unpleasant side effect associated with the first generation of antipsychotics, newer types became developed in the mid-90s. These drugs were referred to as 'second generation antipsychotics', or 'atypical' antipsychotics. Some examples include risperidone; and olanzapine.

Atypical antipsychotics became increasingly prescribed for people with dementia in the late 2000s. However, a report from the Department of Health in 2009 criticised their heavy use, and warned that they gave rise to significant negative side-effects in dementia patients.

Some antipsychotics have been shown to be effective in reducing the intensity of behavioural and psychological symptoms in people with dementia. However, Risperidone is currently the only antipsychotic drug that has been licensed for treatment as a short-term measure for aggression in Alzheimer's' disease, if the aggression is of an intensity where there is a risk of harm to the person or others, and if the person has not responded to other non-drug approaches.

The benefits of antipsychotics are that they can help to reduce symptoms of aggression, or sometimes psychosis. However, they can also give rise to a number of significant drawbacks and risks:

- They can take a lot of time before effects are manifested: sometimes between 6 – 12 weeks;
- If people with Lewy body dementia (which produce visual hallucinations) are prescribed such anti-psychotics, then they must be regularly reviewed, as they may develop particularly severe adverse reactions.
- Other risks include:
    - Sedation or drowsiness;
    - Parkinsonism (shaking and unsteadiness)
    - Worsen physical health; dehydration and water retention; increased likelihood of chest infections; cardiovascular problems.
    - Increased risk of infections: falls; blood clots; stroke; worsening of other dementia symptoms; death.
- Use of antipsychotics always need to be closely monitored and reviewed.
- It has been estimated that antipsychotics cause an additional 1,800 deaths approximately each year. The risk of death increases the longer the patient is taking antipsychotics, particularly if they are taking them for several years.

If other antipsychotic drugs are prescribed for people with dementia, then they are done so 'off-label', which means there must be a very good reason to do so, in accordance with General Medical Council guidelines.

Antipsychotics can only be prescribed in the first instance, by a specialist doctor: such as, a geriatrician, a GP with a speciality in dementia; or an old-age psychiatrist. Any prescription of an antipsychotic medication will be subject to regular review, or a possible gradual reduction in the future.

Risks:

- Antipsychotic drugs can increase the risk of severe adverse reactions in people with Lewy body dementia, or Parkinson's disease dementia, and would therefore need to be prescribed under heightened care and vigilance, and stepped-up supervision and review.

- Such drugs may have limited effect during episodes of care which tend to give rise to repeat symptoms of distress or anxiety. Other approaches are better at responding to anxiety or distress that are caused by specific identifiable triggers.

ANTIDEPRESSANTS

Commonly prescribed for people with dementia, are antidepressants such as: sertraline; citalopram; mirtazapine and trazodone.

While citalopram can help to reduce symptoms of depression, it cannot be used on its own to treat agitation in people with Alzheimer's disease because the high dose of it that would be required for this purpose, would cause significant negative side effects on the person's memory and cardiovascular health.

ANTICONVULSANTS

Anticonvulsants are a group of medications that are used to reduce the frequency of seizures in people with epilepsy.

However, some anticonvulsants have been shown to have effects in reducing aggression and agitation in people with dementia.

One such drug is called, carbamazepine. However, this is only used as an absolute last resort, where other drugs have been shown not to work, as it can give rise to many other negative side effects: such as sedation; falls; skin rashes; blood disorders and low sodium levels.

There has not been much research to prove conclusively the effectiveness of other anticonvulsants, such as gabapentin, for people with dementia. Moreover, some anticonvulsants such as valproate have now been recommended not to be given to reduce agitation or aggression levels in people with dementia.

ANXIETY

Anxiety is a common condition, that many of us experience from time to time. People with dementia may be particularly prone to feeling anxious, due the interference that the disease wreaks on their ability to carry out everyday activities.

Making time for people, providing gentle reassurance and activities to help alleviate anxiety, such as getting some fresh air, going for a walk, or listening to music, can go a long way to helping people with mild anxiety.

Some people have more severe levels of anxiety, which can either manifest every now and then, or be persistent and enduring.

TREATMENTS:

- **Antidepressants:** e.g. sertraline
- **Benzodiazepines:** most effective when used for short periods, of no more than two weeks. If used for longer, then these drugs can become addictive, and give rise to very distressing withdrawal symptoms if the person stops taking them. They can give rise to other side effects, especially in people with dementia, such as: excessive sedation (drowsiness); unsteadiness; increased risk of falls; greater confusion and memory problems.
- **'Z' drugs (non-benzodiazepines):** These drugs are used to treat sleep problems. Their side effects can be similar to benzodiazepines. Examples: zaleplon; zolpidem; zopiclone.
- **Buspirone:** helps to reduce anxiety, but not addictive like benzodiazepines, and does not cause drowsiness. Only recommended to use for short period of time. [xxiv]

SLEEP DISTURBANCES

Sleep disturbances are frequently experienced by people with dementia, and also their carers. There are many different reasons for this. Sometimes sleep disturbances may be a result of the progressive symptoms of the dementia itself. There may also be other factors, however, such as:

- Primary sleep disorders (sleep apnoea; restless legs syndrome);
- Coexisting psychiatric conditions;
- Medication side effects;
- Environmental and behavioural factors;
- ... or a combination of these different factors.

Drug treatments:

- **Sedatives (e.g. benzodiazepines; nonbenzodiazepines):** Are recommended to be used for only a short period of time, as they can give rise to other side effects, such as: daytime sleepiness; anterograde amnesia; confusion.
- **Antidepressants:** possible side effects can include excessive sedation; dizziness; weight gain.
- **Non-drug interventions:** physical exercise; limiting daytime napping; regular routines with regards night-time and morning; avoiding alcohol, nicotine and caffeine; consistent mealtimes; sleep environment being not too hot or cold.[xxv]

PAIN

Pain is a phenomenon that affect many people with dementia, and can have a wide-ranging impact on all areas of life. Pain can be difficult to manage, because there are different types of pain, and finding the underlying cause can be challenging when the person affected is have increasing difficulty in terms of communication.

Pain can give worsen mental health conditions such as anxiety and depression. It can also affect one's physical health, in both indirect and direct ways. Pain can lead to reduced appetite, which then leads to weight loss, frailty, increased risk of falls, and reduced mobility. On the other hand, pain can also affect one's ability to have a good night's sleep: insomnia can further exacerbate memory problems, and also increase mood problems, leading to aggression and agitation.

The effects of untreated, or under-treated, pain is multifaceted, therefore. A person with advanced dementia, may well not be able to communicate their pain, although this makes it all the more important for healthcare practitioners to observe indicators of pain:

- **Physical indicators**: e.g. tooth decay; ear problems; ingrown toenails; pressure areas on the skin.
- **Behavioural changes:** e.g. uncharacteristic behaviours, such as being quieter than usual or refusing to eat; changes in facial expression.
- **Disturbed behaviour:** e.g. increased paranoia; hallucinating; aggression; agitation; increased restlessness; calling out.

Recognition and improving the management of pain for people with dementia is very important, and requires a joined-up approach from different professionals. People need to have regular reviews of their dementia, as well as for other physical and mental health conditions, and behavioural changes. Family and carers should also be involved in the care of the individual as much as possible, because often they know and understand the intricacies of the person better than anyone else, and can pick up on subtle changes quicker.

It is also important to use simple language when talking with a person with dementia about pain. You should use straight-forward words such as 'pain', 'sore', or 'hurt' not complicated, more technical language, such as 'inflammation', 'haemorrhoids' or 'varicose veins'. It is also important to take into consideration a person's cultural, religious or ethnic characteristics, which might influence ideas about when to ask for help to manage pain, or the language used when describing it. There are also a number of pain assessment tools/ scales, that can help a person with communication difficulties, to have their pain assessed:

- Abbey
- DOLOPLUS2
- Pain Assessment Checklist for Seniors with Limited Ability to Communicate (PACSLAC)
- Pain Assessment in Advanced Dementia (PAINAD)
- Disability Distress Assessment Tool (DisDat)

TREATMENT & MANAGEMENT OF PAIN

There is no 'magic bullet' in terms of medication, in terms of the management of long term. A combination of pharmacological and non-pharmacological interventions is necessary, with healthcare practitioners working in a joined-up approach.

There are a number of factors that have to be determined before deciding on the optimum intervention for pain management. These include:

- **The type of pain:** neuropathic; nociceptive; mixed form
- **The underlying cause of the pain:** musculoskeletal; visceral; cancer; neuropathic
- Characteristics of the pain: acute (would require short-acting, pulsatile drugs); chronic (would require sustained-release drugs)
- **Risk:** benefit assessment, with specific considerations for people with dementia:
- falls and/or postural hypotension; sedation; renal impairment
- **Medicine optimisation:** for example, cost versus clinical effectiveness; patient-centred; realistic outcomes; appropriate formulation (buccal; oro-dispersible; transdermal)
- **Proactive management of potential side-effects of opioids:** e.g. pain relief/ laxatives; anti-emetics
- **Formulation:** if the person with dementia has difficulties with swallowing (dysphagia), then alternative formulation for medications should be considered.
- **Regular reviews**: should be conducted to assess the impact and effectiveness of the treatment. The timing and frequency of these reviews will depend on the

intensity and type of pain; the treatment prescribed; the appearance of side-effects; failure to respond to treatment.

Other non-drug approaches should also be considered, such as:

- Acupuncture
- Animal therapy
- Aromatherapy
- Cognitive behaviour therapy
- Exercise
- Music therapy
- Physiotherapy
- Reflexology
- TENS (transcutaneous electrical nerve stimulation)

MEDICATION APPROACHES

Basic principles: 'start low and go slow' and adjust the dose to the effectiveness of response.

NON-OPIOID TREATMENTS

- Paracetamol: this is usually considered the first option for people with acute or chronic pain.
- Anti-depressants
- Anti-epileptics
- NSAIDs

OPIOID TREATMENTS

Recommended to start at the lowest recommended dose, and to proactively manage side-effects like constipation or nausea. There are different formulations available: liquid formulations; oro-dispersible; patches; suppositories; syringe-driven treatments

- Buprenorphine
- Codeine
- Dihydrocodeine

- Fentanyl
- Morphine
- Oxycodone
- Tramadol [xxvi]

'PRN' MEDICATION

'PRN' stands for 'pro re nata', and refers to medications that are only given 'when required', for many different conditions.

Such medication plays an important part in relieving short-term ailments, which if left untreated could worsen underlying conditions.

Here are some examples of conditions that can be relieved with PRN medicines:

- Nausea
- Vomiting
- Pain
- Indigestion
- Anxiety
- Insomnia

There are also some long-term conditions, that can require people to use PRN medicines: such as, people with asthma.

These interventions can go a long way to helping people to manage their own self-care, fluctuating long-term conditions, or short-term difficulties. Such medicines should be offered in a person-centred way, and at the time when they are experiencing symptoms: they should not only be offered during medication rounds, or according to the times printed on MAR sheets. It is important that time the of dosage of such medications is recorded effectively, so that emerging patterns can be identified and assessed, during the person's medication reviews.[xxvii]

IMPORTANCE OF RECORDING AND REPORTING SIDE-EFFECTS

We have seen that dementia often comes accompanied by a host of complicating conditions, like depression or sleep disorders, and dementia is itself composed of many different subtypes of the disease. The management of medication for a person with dementia, should therefore primarily be seen as a dynamic and person-centred process.

With the progressive, debilitating disease that dementia brings, the persons affected often find over time that they cannot comprehend, articulate or communicate the origin, nature or intensity of any pain they may be experiencing.

With the passage of time, the importance of the role of healthcare practitioners to utilise their skills to observe, record and report behavioural or physical signs of pain, and to advocate on behalf of the person with dementia, becomes ever more important.

Too often, the side effects that a person with dementia may be experiencing, such as constipation or sleep difficulties, are simply shrugged off. In fact, it is important to track and monitor all such reported or observed side effects, because it is only after time, and with consistent recording and dedication by a healthcare team, that patterns emerge, and action can then be taken.

There are different medications, formulations, and approaches available to help make the experience of dementia as least distressing as possible for people concerned. It is up to healthcare practitioners to feel the responsibility and potential in their role as advocates, and to exercise their duty of care to the best of their ability.

SUMMARY

Type of Medication	Name/ Brand Name	Therapeutic Effect	Side Effect/ Disadvantages
Medication to reduce dementia symptoms:			
Cholinesterase Inhibitors	Donepezil (aka Aricept); Rivastigmine (aka Exelon); Galantamine (aka Reminyl; Reminyl XL; Acumor XL; Galsya XL & Gatalin XL). (XL means a slow-release form of the drug)	Reduces anxiety; Improves: motivation; memory; concentration; functional abilities.	**Side-Effects:** loss of appetite; nausea; vomiting; diarrhoea; muscle cramps; headaches; dizziness; fatigue; insomnia **Disadvantages:** Benefits certain types of dementia, but not others. Limited effect on environmental/ contextual triggers of agitation and aggression.
NMDA Receptor Antagonists	Memantine (aka Ebixa; Maruxa or Nemdatine)	Positive effects for people with severe levels of dementia; alleviates symptoms of aggression and agitation.	Dizziness; headaches; tiredness; raised blood pressure; constipation.
Other forms of dementia:			
Frontotemporal dementia	Antidepressants		
Vascular dementia	Drugs to treat cardiovascular/ blood pressure conditions.		
Antipsychotics	**First generation/ 'typical' anti-psychotics:** thioridazine;	**Effects:** Alleviates symptoms of aggression and agitation	**Side-effects:** motor control disorders; sedation

	haloperidol; stelazine.		
	Second generation/ 'atypical' anti-psychotics: risperidone; olanzapine.	**Effects:** Alleviates symptoms of aggression and agitation	**Side-effects/ drawbacks:** takes a long time for effects to become apparent; can cause severe adverse reactions in people with Lewy body dementia; can lead to other side effects, such as: sedation/ drowsiness; parkinsonism (shaking and unsteadiness); dehydration; water retention; increased risk of chest infections; cardiovascular problems; falls; blood clots; death.
Antidepressants	**Examples:** sertraline; citalopram; mirtazapine and trazodone.		**Side-effects:** Citalopram cannot be used at high doses to treat AD, as can cause cardiovascular problems.
Anticonvulsants	**Example:** carbamazepine	**Effects:** Helps to reduce aggression and agitation.	**Side-effects:** sedation; falls; skin rashes; blood disorders; low sodium levels.
Anxiety	**Antidepressants:** e.g. sertraline **Benzodiazepines:** Useful for short-term **'Z' drugs (non-benzodiazepines):** e.g. zaleplon; zolpidem; zopiclone. Buspirone: helps to reduce anxiety and less addictive.		Can lead to drowsiness; and not recommended for long term use.

Sleep	**Sedatives** (e.g. benzodiazepines; nonbenzodiazepines):	Recommended for short-term use;	**Side effects:** include daytime sleepiness; anterograde amnesia; confusion.
	Antidepressants:	Helps alleviate sleep problems.	**Side effects:** excessive sedation; dizziness; weight gain.
Pain	**Non-opioid:** paracetamol; anti-depressants; anti-epileptics; NSAIDs		
	Opioid treatments: buprenorphine; codeine; dihydrocodeine; fentanyl; morphine; oxycodone; tramadol.	**Effects:** can help relief pain and secondary effects of un-/undermanaged pain: e.g. reduced appetites; weight loss; frailty; increased risk of falls; reduced mobility; insomnia; memory and mood problems.	**Side-effects/ disadvantages:** can lead to increased risk of falls and/or postural hypotension; sedation; renal impairment.

Apply and Demonstrate

You have learnt about the range of medications that are used to treat the symptoms, and co-existing conditions (such as depression; aggression and agitation; cognitive function and memory problems; anxiety; sleep disturbance; pain), that commonly feature with dementia.

The Dementia Care Certificate will require you to be able to explain why antipsychotic drugs are used, to relay some examples, but most importantly to show an understanding of the contrasting risks versus their benefits. You will also have to write about the importance of recording and recording these side effects or any adverse reactions.

CHAPTER 7: UNDERSTAND MENTAL WELL-BEING AND MENTAL HEALTH PROMOTION

Personal thoughts and emotions of sadness, fear, trauma or anger, let alone personal experiences from life that can be either positive or traumatic, are deeply sensitive and private.

However, dementia muddles the senses, and one's ability to orientate oneself in time and space. Those memories are still there, sometimes in distorted form in the guise of hallucinations, or harboured in nightmares, but the ability to communicate about them becomes ever more elusive. Opportunities, be there an impromptu conversation or planned activity, to tap into memories, whether small or profound, can help to reignite a sense of personhood and uniqueness.

Superficially, it is the outward behaviour, personality traits or the formalities of diagnoses of people with dementia that concentrate minds of healthcare practitioners. However, finding an outlet for a person, in their own way, time or pace to express, reveal or explore ideas, feelings, or experiences can often be more profound than talking therapies, let alone medication, in helping them both to explore inbuilt feelings, as well as expanding the understanding about them from others.

There are many different forms of creativity, and ways to help people to use creative mediums to find either a form of expression, or simply a form of solace. Some links to websites with ideas and advice about creative therapies, are given at the end of this chapter.

In this section, we will look at just one type of activity that can be adapted as an individual or a group-based exercise, and that is collage art. A collage is essentially a piece of art that is made simply by sticking different materials, such as photographs or cuttings from magazines, fabric or paper, on to a backing. It is a great exercise as it is easily adaptable to circumstances, for example:

- It can be a project that can be worked on over a period of time: can help people with restlessness, short concentration span or low confidence;
- One can encourage the involvement of other service users in the project, which can help to give a sense of community, shared endeavour and ownership over the final piece;

- The activity itself can also be adapted to involve different fabrics which can provide sensory stimulation: such as different textures; fabrics; shapes.

SUGGESTIONS FOR A COLLAGE PROJECT

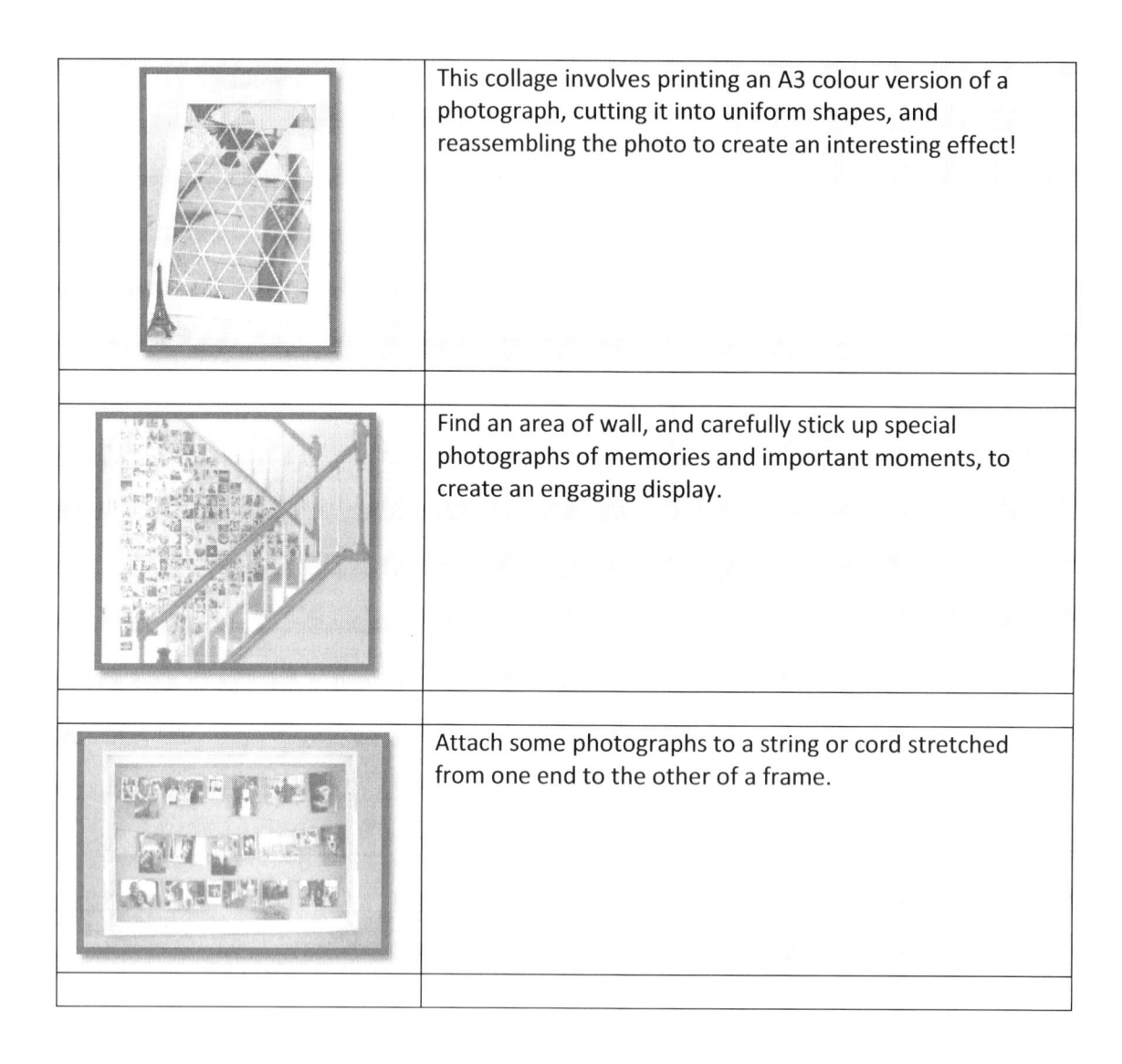

	This collage involves printing an A3 colour version of a photograph, cutting it into uniform shapes, and reassembling the photo to create an interesting effect!
	Find an area of wall, and carefully stick up special photographs of memories and important moments, to create an engaging display.
	Attach some photographs to a string or cord stretched from one end to the other of a frame.

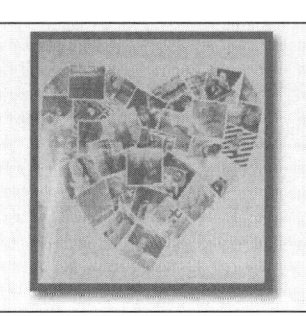

	Attach photographs together on a backing, or wall, in the shape of a heart.

Collages are a great way to encourage activity, creativity and camaraderie along the way. There are many other simple activities that are straightforward to organise, and that can be stimulating but not too challenging for people with dementia. For example:

- Colouring in pictures with pen or colouring pencil;
- Threading colourful beads on thread to create simple bracelets or necklaces;
- Painting;
- Sand art: filling different shaped plastic containers with layers of different coloured sand;
- Mosaic art: using simple adhesive mosaic squares to create artistic designs.

Here are some other websites, where you can garner more ideas and inspiration for other creative activities:

Mind disorders.com: http://www.minddisorders.com/Br-Del/Creative-therapies.html

Mind.org.uk: https://www.mind.org.uk/information-support/drugs-and-treatments/arts-and-creative-therapies/types-of-arts-and-creative-therapies/#.XPV5a4hKjIU

IMPORTANCE OF INVOLVEMENT AND ENGAGEMENT

Helping to carry out a creative activity with an individual or group of service users should be fun and relaxed. If a person does not want to join in, then it's important not to pressure them. If they want to join in for just a few minutes and then stop, then that is absolutely fine. Equally, if they prefer to watch others or just to share the companionship, while others participate, that is also fine if that is what the individual wants to.

Some service users may have less confidence than others, or may prefer to do activities on their own as opposed to in a group. There might be personality conflicts between service users within the group. Or at times, there may be practical barriers to joining in the activity, such as if they struggle with dexterity problems or short attention span.

Talking and camaraderie during a creative exercise is often as important as the activity itself. One could talk about the textures of the materials being used, details in a photograph or ideas that could spark a memory of a person, place or experience from a long time ago. Of course, there are times when the best kind of talking is silence: if a service user appears to want, or asks for silence, or if they struggle to manage too much sensory stimulation, it is better to minimise the amount one is talking oneself, or initiating the conversation.

However, engaging verbally in a way that is appropriate to the preferences and needs of the service users, also helps one to gauge their perception of the activity, and if you need to make any adaptations to it. Talking to them can help you to deduce what they have gained from the activity – a sense of purpose; a sense of keeping busy; or doing something enjoyable. You can gauge how you might need to tweak the activity to make it easier to set up, or replicated by other staff members, or make it more accessible next time.

You should always record any insights or findings that are discovered as a result of doing activities with service users with dementia: for example, finding out a type of music that an individual is passionate about, or evokes a special memory; changing difficulties with hand-eye coordination, which might suggest progression of their dementia symptoms; or if a particular activity gives a person a sense of happiness or wellbeing, this can give others ideas of similar activities they could do with that individual as well. If information isn't shared, it is only useful in that moment. If relevant information is shared and in an appropriate way, to improve the compassion and quality of care provided to people with dementia, then it becomes transformative.

Apply and Demonstrate

You now have the ideas and knowledge to be able to carry out your own collage, or other creative, activity with a service user or group, within the care setting where you work.

STRATEGIES FOR MENTAL HEALTH

NO HEALTH WITHOUT MENTAL HEALTH (2011)

The Government launched the strategy, with the aim to create 'parity of esteem' between physical and mental health, across the whole range of health, social care and other local services. The objective of the strategy was also to improve mental health for all, and to increase the quality and effectiveness of mental health services[xxviii].

SUMMARY OF OBJECTIVES OF THE STRATEGY:

- More people will have good mental health
- More people with mental health problems will recover
- More people with mental health problems will have good physical health
- More people will have a positive experience of care and support
- Fewer people will suffer avoidable harm
- Fewer people will experience stigma and discrimination

WHAT IS MENTAL HEALTH?

Mental health is about wellbeing, which isn't just about medications to address symptoms. It is also about being able to make the most of opportunities through life, being supported to overcome obstacles and to achieve personal fulfilment: 'starting well, developing well, working well, living well and ageing well'.

Implicit within this interpretation of mental health, is the following framework of what is meant by the term 'recovery', which means:

- **Hope:** ensuring that it is possible for people to pursue their personal goals and ambitions;
- **Control:** helping people to maintain a sense of control over their lives;
- **Opportunity:** supporting people to build their lives beyond mental illness.

RESPONSIBILITIES OF LOCAL AUTHORITIES:

- To appoint an elected member as 'mental health champion'
- To assess how their strategies, commissioning decisions and directly provided services support and improve mental health and wellbeing: including all forms of services, such as housing, planning, transport, leisure and green spaces and other community services.
- To involve the local community, people affected by mental health problems, as well as their families and carers, in help in the coproduction of service design. This should include proactive outreach to 'hard-to-reach' groups, and support for people with communication difficulties to express their views.
- To use the Local Government Association's Knowledge Hub: which allows members and staff to share ideas and innovative approaches in the context of mental health services.
- Sign up to the Time to Change campaign: to address the issue of stigma about mental health amongst staff, and raise awareness and understanding of mental health across the county.

RECOMMENDATIONS FOR ADULT SOCIAL SERVICES AND CHILDREN'S SERVICES

- To use community care and carers assessments to identify ways to support independence and promote recovery;
- To work alongside CCGs to remodel existing support to focus on early intervention, service integration, personalisation and recovery;
- To provide individual budgets and direct payments for people with mental health problems;
- To work alongside CCGs, schools and wider children's services to focus on early intervention and integrated support;
- To offer evidence-based parenting interventions to families with children at risk of conduct disorder
- To improve emotional support for looked after and adopted children and care leavers
- To support schemes and services that promote positive parenting, and supports at risk families.

CONCLUSION

I hope this book has been stimulating reading, has widened your knowledge, understanding about dementia and also supports your studies and coursework towards attainment of the Dementia Care Certificate.

More importantly, I hope this book will increase your passion and energy for supporting people with dementia, who are not just 'people with dementia', but precious individuals with immense experience, value, creativity and uniqueness.

REFERENCES

[i] Headway.org.uk. (2019). *About the brain*. [online] Available at: https://www.headway.org.uk/about-brain-injury/further-information/about-the-brain/ [Accessed 2019].

[ii] England: NHS Digital; Recorded Dementia Diagnosis Data August 2018. Wales: General medical services contract: Quality and outcomes framework 2017/18. Scotland: Information Services Division; Quality and Outcomes Framework General Practice. Northern Ireland: Department of Health; 2017/18 raw disease prevalence trend data for Northern Ireland.

[iii] Prince, M et al (2014) Dementia UK: Update Second Edition report produced by King's College London and the London School of Economics for the Alzheimer's Society.

[iv] Prince, M et al (2014): Update Second Edition report produced by King's College London and the London School of Economics for the Alzheimer's Society.

[v] Lewis et al (2014). Trajectory of Dementia in the UK – Making a Difference, report produced by the Office of Health Economics for Alzheimer's Research UK.

[vi] Lakey, L. (2009) Counting the cost: Caring for people with dementia on hospital wards published by the Alzheimer's Society.

[vii] Etkind, S.N. et al (2017) How many people will need palliative care in 2040? Past trends, future projections and implications for services. BMC Medicine 2017 15:102.

[viii] Dowrick, A. Southern, A. (2014). Dementia 2014: Opportunity for change by the Alzheimer's Society.

[ix] Dementia Statistics Hub. (2019). *Dementia Statistics Hub | Alzheimer's Research UK*. [online] Available at: https://www.dementiastatistics.org [Accessed 2019].

[x] Scie.org.uk. (2019). *Dementia risk factors - SCIE*. [online] Available at: https://www.scie.org.uk/dementia/symptoms/diagnosis/risk-factors.asp?gclid=CjwKCAjwiN_mBRBBEiwA9N-e_gr8MYQA-boGKldEzzGTmEolSzqY1z6HUrByfw9dmkER60vkyZVy1RoCZ00QAvD_BwE [Accessed 2019].

[xi] "The MMSE Test." *Alzheimer's Society*, www.alzheimers.org.uk/about-dementia/symptoms-and-diagnosis/diagnosis/mmse-test.

[xii] Human-memory.net. (2019). *Types of Memory - The Human Memory*. [online] Available at: http://www.human-memory.net/types.html [Accessed 2019].

[xiii] Mcleod, Saul. "Skinner - Operant Conditioning." *B.F. Skinner | Operant Conditioning | Simply Psychology*, Simply Psychology, 28 Jan. 2018, www.simplypsychology.org/operant-conditioning.html.

[xiv] "Delusional Disorder and Types of Delusions: Symptoms, Causes, Diagnosis, Treatment." *WebMD*, WebMD, www.webmd.com/schizophrenia/guide/delusional-disorder#1.

[xv] GOV.UK. (2019). *Definition of disability under the Equality Act 2010*. [online] Available at: https://www.gov.uk/definition-of-disability-under-equality-act-2010 [Accessed 2019].

[xvi] Oxford Dictionaries | English. (2019). *relationship | Definition of relationship in English by Oxford Dictionaries*. [online] Available at: https://en.oxforddictionaries.com/definition/relationship [Accessed 2019].

[xvii] Zilkens, R. R., Bruce, D. G., Duke, J., Spilsbury, K., & Semmens, J. B. (2014). Severe psychiatric disorders in mid-life and risk of dementia in late- life (age 65-84 years): a population based case-control study. *Current Alzheimer research, 11*(7), 681-93.

[xviii] de Vries PJ, Honer WG, Kemp PM, et al. Dementia as a complication of schizophrenia. Journal of Neurology, Neurosurgery & Psychiatry 2001;70:588-596.

[xix] Moll, A. (2013). Losing track of time. Dementia and the ageing prison population: treatment challenges and examples of good practice. Mental Health Foundation.

[xx] "Prison Care Pathways for Older Offenders in Prisons." East of England CLAHRC, 13 Sept. 2018, www.clahrc-eoe.nihr.ac.uk/2016/07/prison-care-pathways/.

[xxi] Alzheimer's Society. (2019). *Effects of Alzheimer's disease drugs*. [online] Available at: https://www.alzheimers.org.uk/about-dementia/treatments/drugs/effects-of-alzheimers-drugs [Accessed 2019].

[xxii] Scie.org.uk. (2019). *Antipsychotic medication and dementia - SCIE*. [online] Available at: https://www.scie.org.uk/dementia/living-with-dementia/difficult-situations/antipsychotic-medication.asp [Accessed 2019].

[xxiii] Porter-Brooks, S. (2019). *Understanding Schizoaffective Disorder*. UK: Independently published, pp.23-31.

[xxiv] Alzheimer's Society. (2019). *Effects of Alzheimer's disease drugs*. [online] Available at: https://www.alzheimers.org.uk/about-dementia/treatments/drugs/effects-of-alzheimers-drugs [Accessed 2019].

[xxv] Deschenes, Cynthia L, and Susan M McCurry. "Current treatments for sleep disturbances in individuals with dementia." *Current psychiatry reports* vol. 11,1 (2009): 20-6. doi:10.1007/s11920-009-0004-2

[xxvi] Guidelines. (2019). *Pain management in dementia guideline*. [online] Available at: https://www.guidelines.co.uk/pain/pain-management-in-dementia-guideline/250682.article [Accessed 2019].

[xxvii] Cqc.org.uk. (2019). *When required (PRN) medicines | Care Quality Commission*. [online] Available at: https://www.cqc.org.uk/guidance-providers/adult-social-care/when-required-prn-medicines [Accessed 2019].

[xxviii] Mind.org.uk. (2019). [online] Available at: https://www.mind.org.uk/media/343118/No_Health_Without_Mental_Health_Local_Authorities.pdf [Accessed 2019].

OTHER BOOKS BY THIS AUTHOR:

Leadership and Management in Health and Social Care, and Children and Young Peoples' Services: *The down-to-earth learner support guide.*

Understanding Autism and Positive Behavioural Support

Understanding Dementia: *A friendly and accessible companion reader for professionals, families and people affected by dementia*

To Be Invisible: *Unveiling the truth about eating disorders*

Level 3 Diploma for Children and Young People's Workforce: A comprehensive learner support guide

Printed in Great Britain
by Amazon